Foods Four Tho̵ ̵t

Four Food Groups to Repair Your Child's Gut and Improve
Symptoms of Autism, ADHD and Autoimmune Disorders

by Crystal Jordan, B.I.S.

Foods Four Thought Diet

Four Food Groups to Repair Your Child's Gut and Improve Symptoms of Autism, ADHD and Autoimmune Disorders

Published by Foods Four Thought, LLC
Copyright © 2021 by Crystal Jordan
ISBN 978-0-578-85613-1
First Printing, 2021

All rights reserved. No part of this book may be reproduced in any form by any electronic or mechanical means including information storage and retrieval systems—except in the case of brief quotations in articles or reviews—without the permission in writing from its publisher, Crystal Jordan.

www.foodsfourthought.com

Dedication

This book is a work of love, and is humbly dedicated to my children. You have given this life of mine purpose and beauty. And to my husband, my soul's companion. You have helped me see all that I am.

This book presents the research and ideas of its author. It is not intended to be a substitute for consultation with a professional healthcare practitioner. Consult with your healthcare practitioner before starting any diet or supplement regimen. The publisher and author disclaim responsibility for any adverse effects resulting directly or indirectly from the information contained in this book.

Content

Chapter 1 — Welcome 1
    What You Will Find in This Book 3
    A Word of Wisdom 5

Chapter 2 — A Story of Healing: Our Personal Journey 9

Chapter 3 — The Science of Dysfunction and Digestion 19
    Effects of Pathogens 20
    The Power of Bacteria and Fungus 22
    The Brain-Gut Connection 24
    Carbohydrate Reaction 26
    The Trouble with GFCF 27
    The Autoimmune Link 28

                                                             29
    How the Diet Works 31
    How Long Does the Diet Take to Work? 33
    Journal Everything 34
    My Child Doesn't Have GI Problems. Will the Diet Still Help? 35

Chapter 5 — All About Food 37
    What Not to Eat and Why 37
    What You Can Eat 43
    Introducing Foods Later 51
    Supplements 51
    Foods Four Thought vs. Other Diets 55

Chapter 6 — Communication 57
    Interactive Menu 58
    Interactive Health Checklist 59
    Interactive Calendar Goal 60

Chapter 7 — Ready to Begin 63
    Setting a Start Date 63
    Clear Your Cupboards 64
    Going Shopping 65
    The Meal Plan 67
    Meal Prep 68

Chapter 8 — Phases of the Diet 73
    Phase One: Weeks 1–2, Getting Started 73
    Phase Two: Weeks 3–8, Keep it Going 80
    Phase Three: Weeks 9+, Reintroduction 84

Chapter 9 — Additional Tools 91
    Planning for Parties and School 91
    Organization 95
    Overcoming Obstacles and Negativity 97
    Self-Care 99

Chapter 10 — A Final Word 103

Chapter 11 — In the Kitchen and Recipes 105
    Glycemic Index of Fruit 105
    Substitution Chart 106
    Kitchen Must-Haves 108
    1-Week Shopping List 110
    1-Week Meal Plan 117
    Recipes for the 1-Week Meal Plan 119
        Breakfast 121
        Lunch & Snacks 135
        Dinner 148
        Sweet Treats 179
    Allowed and Non-Permitted Food List 193

Additional Resources 235
References 244
Index 254

CHAPTER 1

WELCOME

I feel as though I know you. Your struggle, your pain, your worry, and your unwavering love through it all. I have been there; I am still there. As parents, we live in this space. The fine balance of pure joy and heartache, of triumph and disappointment. Our adult lives now revolve around ensuring our children get every positive drop and morsel this world has to offer them.

If you're parenting a child with unique needs, this book is written for you. Together, you and I will discuss why diet is the most powerful approach to help your child. The pages ahead specifically address autism spectrum disorder (ASD), attention deficit hyperactivity disorder (ADHD), and autoimmune disorders. I will also help you successfully implement this program in your home, even if you have a picky eater. The diet's guidelines will also more than likely optimize your own health. Thus, amongst other reasons, I highly recommend the dietary rules be followed by all family members.

As a parent of a child with distinct needs, be they physical or behavioral, your life is undoubtedly filled with daily challenges. Undertaking new ventures with your child can be exciting, scary, and difficult all wrapped up into one. Changes are always hard, especially for our kids who often crave consistency and predictability. In your home this may look like dry crunchy food, yogurt with no chunks, all things circular, tagless shirts, or shorts in the winter. I get it. I and many others have been there too, this new place that you are preparing to venture. A journey that involves you getting your family to become part of a healthful way of living. We have successfully gotten through it and you will too.

The Foods Four Thought Diet, or FFT Diet, that lies ahead may be the greatest step you will take towards your child's best health. And while this diet will have an end—that being the healing of their intestinal tract, followed by better physical and mental health—I heartily suggest that as you move through all steps of the diet, you do so with a mind towards a healthier lifestyle now and forever after. This means you continue to opt for meal planning and preparation over delivery pizza ninety-five percent of the time. That you stick to the produce isles over the boxes and cans at the grocery store. Plan on maintaining your newfound way of eating healthy and teach your child what nutritious foods look and feel like after being eaten—so as they grow older, they too can make good decisions about food. This will allow them to maintain their best health throughout their lifetime.

Improving your child's physical, behavioral, and emotional wellness starts by changing the food you put on their plate day in and day out. This challenge is a matter of taking it one day at a time. If followed completely, you will have corrected their digestive issues, boosted their immune system, improved sleep patterns, energy levels, behaviors, and so much more. You will have enhanced their quality of life, thus yours as well. And believe me, the more positive changes you experience because of the diet, the more motivation you will feel to continue and make this lifestyle change work.

What You Will Find in This Book

First, I'll walk you through our story and how we found ourselves avid believers that diet is the most powerful intervention. We will then discuss the science behind the disorders discussed in this book and why certain individuals are at particular risk of having digestive and autoimmune problems. We'll learn how the gut and brain interact with each other and why the health of the intestine is critical to the health of the brain and body. This is a very important section that will help instill a strong *why* to the diet. Understanding what is occurring within the body beyond much of our vision will encourage you to stick to the guidelines.

We will also address what the Foods Four Thought Diet is and what foods can and cannot be eaten. We'll learn how to plan for the diet and communicate with your family about the changes ahead. For many, this element of teamwork and communication is the most difficult part. Getting your child, siblings, significant other, grandparents, and teachers to get on board with the dietary changes is a monumental task. If you are concerned about your child's lack of communication skills, don't be. This is addressed and will be supported. Having them take part in the process of eating healthy is so important, I have thus provided several tools to support these changes. Finally, we will discuss meal planning, organization, and self-care.

If you're already nervous because you don't feel comfortable cooking, don't be. The recipes in this book are delicious and simple. Meaning they can be placed in a single pot or cooker and ready in 30 minutes, or thrown into a blender, then into the oven and, presto! Dinner is served. There are only a few ingredients to always keep on hand. With these, you will always have delicious and healthy food at your fingertips. The recipes are also often designed to be large enough that you can keep leftovers for another meal, minimizing your stress levels and time in the kitchen. Plus, the recipes included are intended to appeal to sensory needs and finicky eaters. Lastly, to help you get started, you will be equipped with a 1-week meal plan and shopping guide.

I'll reiterate once again that as you prepare to embark on this new venture, you are not alone. I was once where you are now—pursuing uncharted and intimidating territory. It won't be perfect. You will learn, change, and adapt as you move forward. Just do your best to stay the course. Celebrate even the smallest victories. Maintain a positive mentality. Be patient with yourself and your child because these big changes take time.

A Word of Wisdom

The Foods Four Thought Diet, or any other treatment for that matter, is not intended to "cure" our children, particularly if their challenge is neurological. However, it will absolutely provide the best opportunity for the health and functioning of our incredible kids. Our neuro-diverse children do not need to be cured. They need our attention, love, and positive energy to help them obtain their best level of health. And given their inclined internal sensitivities, this will take greater effort on your part.

Though often difficult, my son's autism has been the greatest gift he could have given me. If you are at the beginning of your voyage and your child is still very young, this may be hard to understand. The early years can be the most difficult and lonely if you have a little one that is wired differently. But having a child who needs you so completely to learn and understand this bustling world is a wonderfully humbling and testing thing. When my son was very young, I wanted to "fix" him entirely. I wanted him to stride out from his bedroom and appropriately ask me what was for breakfast. And while that didn't happen within the time frame I originally had in mind; he is on track to becoming the best possible version of himself this life has to offer.

In the early parts of our journey, I recall encountering so many books, blogs, or videos that described parents of once-autistic children who were now completely "normal." Whether those were accurate or not, I can't be sure, but they were what I was aiming toward and measuring much progress up against. And while I am all for endeavoring towards the highest level of achievement, it is also equally imperative to strike a balance between striving and contentment. To find joy within the present. To set goals but not be devastated if they don't come to pass within your expected timeline. To appreciate the difficulty and recognize that amidst breaking you down, your trials are also building you up. This can often seem impossible when you feel you are inside the eye of a tornado. But maintaining the knowledge that you will come out so much wiser and better is imperative.

Having a mindset that is too focused on maximum achievement will prevent you from enjoying your child, your family, or yourself to the highest level. Trust me, I know, because

I ventured through that dark space of longing. I wanted something that I didn't have and had no idea of how to get it. It wasn't until I created the clearing that allowed me to see all of the joy and development happening right before my eyes.

Like all diversities, autism, ADHD, and autoimmune disorders are a gift. I am not saying this as a manic optimist. It is a simple truth. For those who manage high-functioning mental and behavioral challenges, their creativity, perspective of the world, or unique ability to specialize has helped bring our development as a society to the point it is today. Those on the lower end of functional ability also bring great light to this world. They provide us the opportunity to see humankind with compassion, and a level of unconditional love that is difficult to come by without knowing such individuals. Autoimmune disorders also provide opportunities for growth despite their difficulty. They lend us and our children strength, knowledge, and empathy.

Knowing and loving someone with a disorder provides the immeasurable gift of having greater compassion towards people as a whole. Understanding a dysfunction forces us to reconcile the undeniable reality that we cannot judge people we come in contact with. We are all far too unique and we can't know the struggle someone else faces despite their apparent normalcy.

It is my sincere desire that this book brings light to you and a deepened knowledge of nutrition and the role it plays for all of us, particularly our children with unique needs. The truth is, without proper nutrition, we become less. Less capable of reaching our ultimate physical and mental ability. Therefore, an appreciation for what we put into our and our family's bodies should be considered a top priority in our daily lives.

I am your ally and have traveled this path. Others have done the same. Thus, I know you too can take this critical challenge and make it an imperative part of your life. My warmest wishes are with you from this moment and onward as you move through your journey.

CHAPTER 2

A STORY OF HEALING: OUR PERSONAL JOURNEY

As a child I dreamed of having a massive family, nine kids to be exact. Though, I would later realize I wasn't even close to being mother-to-9-kids-material. My husband and I met when I least expected it. I had recently sworn off dating altogether when he strolled into my life. We had been reluctantly set up on a blind date, yet all it took was that first meeting to realize we were a perfect match. Our courtship was easy and seamless. So much so, it only lasted four and a half months before we were blissfully married. Marriage continued to be a new and fun adventure. We'd stay up late watching Jack Bauer in episodes of *24* while eating bottomless bowls of cereal. It was perfect, but this level of simplicity was short-lived. Six weeks after we were married, I became pregnant. Not exactly part of the plan as it was about two years too soon, but this was happening. It was real, and mental adjustments would have to be made. We accepted our new but exciting reality that life had dealt us with thorough and dutiful preparation.

As with all expecting parents, the months leading up to our first-born's arrival were a wonderful flurry of emotions and questions. Like any studious mother-to-be, I had completely consumed *What to Expect When You're Expecting* and had already started marking up *What to Expect the First Year*. We were as ready as we would ever be. It had been a rather seamless pregnancy with only mild nausea in the first trimester. This being our first child, paired with my affinity for planning, learning the gender was an absolute no-brainer. We were elated to learn that our firstborn would be a boy. This seemed perfect for my husband and me as he had been a decorated basketball athlete into college. Passing on the skills, knowledge, and dedication that he had been brought up with just seemed right.

When the due date finally rolled around, it would be only a few more days, a few spicy burritos, and a few long walks later before our little man arrived as a long-limbed, eight-pound embodiment of perfection. It was thrilling. I felt that this life had been custom-built for me. Our newborn was calm for those first few days in the hospital. However, there was a sudden and stabbing shift that occurred on the day we were to pack up and head home. He cried ceaselessly and for no apparent reason. This crying continued throughout the entire following night and for many nights afterward. It was enough to make a young and once optimistic mother wonder what in the world she had gotten herself into. As our sweet baby continued to have many sleepless nights, inevitably my husband and I did too. We attributed his crying and discomfort to colic as this is a common reality for many babies. The long nights were filled with pacing in front of the fireplace, patting his tiny back, and trying to calm the painfully uncomfortable child. We felt helpless but continued to do all we could from gripe water to 3 a.m. car rides—all to soothe his discomfort.

However, despite the topsy-turvy schedule we all endured, our beautiful baby was still a tiny miracle in the perfect way only new life can be. He was sweet, mild-tempered, and a wonderful napper. However, this latter attribute was likely due to an underlying challenge. He was consistently wide awake and ready to take on the world all night long—every night for nearly his entire first year of life. We followed all the textbook suggestions, keeping lights and sounds low for nighttime feedings and even trying to evade naps all together to get him "back on schedule," but nothing worked. It was probably a good thing that we didn't yet know his ability to sleep reasonably through the night would be challenged until he was three years old.

Also, like any half-enthralled, half-anxious parent, I was a vigilant Baby Center subscriber, reading thoroughly every article that might pertain to our new baby. Thus, I was inevitably and fretfully aware of each missed milestone within his first few months of life. One of the earliest markers they tell you to look for is the ability for a baby to lift their head, followed by their ability to roll over, sit up, and crawl—all leading up to that prestigious moment when they take their first steps. None of these took place at the time, or anywhere even close to when they were "supposed" to. He was late to this gross motor party that I felt all other babies had under lockdown. This I took personally. No way was there anything the matter with him. It had to be a total reflection on my inability to be a decent parent, despite my all-in mentality to the realm of parenthood. I spoke with our pediatrician who told us to just wait it out and that some children were in fact just late to the party. This brought me a light sense of comfort. I reassured myself that it made sense. He was pretty laid back after all. This definitely had to be the reason.

Finally, at nearly two years old, he walked. It was such a momentous occasion that I remember it vividly. Within his timeline, he managed to pull all of his weight up and with great uncertainty balance atop his two chunky legs. He then carefully tottered over to a brightly colored blow-up ball pit and retrieved one of many soft plastic balls. It was a wondrous moment.

Because of his delay, we were able to take advantage of a local early intervention organization. Through this, he was provided an occupational and physical therapist, both of which would come to our home once a week for 30–60 minutes. They would prescribe ideas to help him "feel" his world better than he could do on his own. Their recommendations were practical and noninvasive, and we dutifully implemented them along with anything and everything else that seemed appropriate to help fill the gaps. He was still too young to receive any real diagnosis, but words and titles would often emerge from the therapist's lips. These were new to me but included sensory processing disorder, pervasive developmental disorder, and autism.

We recognized too as time passed that this budding child also lacked proper and recommended communication skills, such as forming words and short sentences to express his needs and wants. Thus, we all learned a bit of sign language and our son picked up on it quickly. We even became well versed in the art of distinguishing what his "duh's" meant depending on the enthusiasm behind the sound and the direction his chunky little finger pointed.

Within this time we also used many forms of therapy, from traditional to alternative. Outside of the early intervention therapists, he also did equestrian therapy, nutrigenomics, aromatherapy, and any gadget that promised a "remedy." We also frequented an alternative medicine practitioner who specialized in autism, plus traditional pediatric doctors including a neurologist, geneticist, and gastroenterologist. These therapies ranged from pleasant to more invasive, from affordable to *let's take a second mortgage out on the home* expensive, and from modest results to none at all. But we were new parents who had lived "normal" lives with "normal" opportunities. We wanted desperately for our only child to have these same possibilities in his life as we had in ours. To be successful in school, both academically and socially. To choose any vocation that strikes passion and to make a decent living at it. To have romantic relationships and the prospect of starting a family. We were going to do our part as we saw it to help our son get where he needed to be to attain these things that we had found value in within our lives.

Like most kids with suspected autism, stimulatory behavior became standard for him. Other challenging behavioral symptoms followed, such as lack of proper emotional control. This included him crying unconditionally when there was no actual need to cry, which became a looming yet unforeseeable threat. One such occurrence included absolute ballistics in a shopping cart while I, the hapless parent, had no choice but to conclude our shopping trip. Onlookers stared in amazement, or perhaps disgust as they formed their opinions of the situation. Another form of emotional oddity was his laughing for no apparent reason at the most inappropriate moments. One I vividly recall was during a somber gathering amidst a large group of people. That was fun. Both happened regularly enough that I became anxious about leaving the house for fear of what social discomfort might await.

From around two years of age, our son also experienced regular diarrhea. This made life uncomfortable for him and potty training impossible. At around two-and-a-half years old, his pediatrician recommended he be placed on a gluten-free and casein-free diet. This was then adhered to for one-and-a-half years. However, during this time no significant improvements in his behaviors nor digestive problems were remedied through the GFCF diet alone.

At nearly four years of age, his health was deteriorating. Besides regular diarrhea, his symptoms also grew to include gray colored skin, dark circles under his eyes, teeth that were growing in yellow, and fingernails that were peeling in layers from the top down. This all led to an awareness that he was malnourished despite reasonable nutrients that were included in his current diet. His body was somehow not accepting these incoming vitamins and minerals. It was apparent that a drastic change needed to occur, and so far all the doctors we had seen had been of no significant help.

However, through research and a touch of inspiration, we found the SCD diet, or Specific Carbohydrate Diet. Based on the research it made sense that this would be the appropriate next step towards our son's improved health. It felt right and shed light on the possibility that this protocol just might heal the inner workings of his digestive system and improve externally manifested problems such as diarrhea and even behavioral issues.

It was settled. We had found our answer and started the introduction phase of the diet the very next day. Within two short weeks of strictly adhering to the guidelines of the SCD diet—plus a few of our own based on other research—nearly all of our son's previously problematic health symptoms had vanished. His skin coloring returned to normal, the dark circles completely disappeared, his bowel movements found normalcy, and his fingernails slowly began to rebuild. Besides the remedied external symptoms, his mood swings became less severe, and he started to speak in three-word sentences. This was coming from a previously nonverbal child. It was an incredible turn of events within such a short amount of time and a testament that the healing provided through the right kind of diet was exactly what his body and brain needed. Through the elimination of specific carbohydrates and other inflammatory foods, his body was able to reset and find a new homeostatic level which then allowed healing to begin.

The rest is now history for our son. This wholesome diet eliminated stress on his body and allowed it to heal from the inside out. Years later we continue to adhere primarily to the guidelines you will find in this book because this type of diet allows the body to function optimally. In addition, our son can now enjoy certain treats during parties or events without the side effects he once experienced because the diet allowed his body to rest, reset, and rebuild. He can now thrive to the best of his personal ability, both physically and mentally. And while this story of healing is incredible, it does not stand alone among children diagnosed with autism, ADHD, or various autoimmune disorders. Many others have also benefited by adhering to comparable elimination diets.

And I'll reiterate again; we are not setting out to cure our children, we are here to assist them in finding their best, happiest, and healthiest self. I mentioned earlier that when our son was very young we wanted him to have the same life experiences we had; groups of friends, athletic trophies, a prom, a job. Thankfully we came to recognize that each person's life must take on its own unique course, and that is a wonderful thing. Our son has and will continue to pave his own path in this life. And though it differs from the one my husband and I experienced, it is no less. This is a healthy and liberating mindset, it just takes a moment to warm up to and accept.

I am one hundred percent confident that nutrition is the most important thing we can do for our health, no matter the challenge that faces us. If you step back and look at that for a moment, it makes sense. We are literally putting items in our mouth, swallowing them, and our body is processing and using whatever that item is. The more natural and nutrient-rich, the easier and more efficiently the body can use that item. We'll explore the science of this further in the next chapter, as we gain a deeper understanding of *why* this diet works.

Foods Four Thought Diet

CHAPTER 3

THE SCIENCE OF DYSFUNCTION AND DIGESTION

Developmental disabilities and autoimmune disorders have grown exponentially over the past several decades. Many researchers claim to not entirely understand why these dysfunctions have grown so rapidly. Some suggest that much of the increase is due to improved screening tools. And while this may be partially true, another fact is profoundly certain. There is a strong correlation between each disorder and genetic factors. Additionally, there is a great deal of speculation about how specific genes may be triggered by environmental components, such as genetically engineered food, pollutants, chemical exposure, heavy metals, and a host of other conjectured possibilities.

Effects of Pathogens

Often, ASD and ADHD diagnoses are paired with several adverse health and behavioral symptoms. These may include difficulties with social interaction, impaired communication, repetitive behaviors, short attention span, and intellectual differences that can be positive or difficult. Autoimmune disorders share common physical health challenges such as sleep abnormality, eczema, rashes, and gastrointestinal disturbance. In fact, many studies have established that children who have any one of these diagnoses experience significantly more frequent and severe digestive problems than their typical peers.

The reason for these gastrointestinal challenges can vary but are often linked to an excess of intestinal bacteria and fungi. An overgrowth of these pathogens has been widely researched and found to cause unfavorable neurological effects and health problems to their infected host. These disorder-inducing microorganisms can alter brain chemistry and behaviors linked to anxiety, depression, and even symptoms often exhibited in patients with autism and ADHD. Physical problems also arise under the circumstance of an intestinal overgrowth and can include abdominal discomfort, diarrhea, constipation, fatigue, skin disturbance, weakened immune response, and the list goes on.

These manifested issues may be due to the disrupted intestinal integrity within the small intestine caused by the overgrowth of bacteria and fungi. This then leads to what is commonly known as leaky gut, followed by malabsorption of nutrients along with digestive and physiological problems.

The importance of intestinal integrity is displayed through a multitude of studies conducted on animals and humans. One assessment included mice that were induced with colitis, an intestinal disorder that often leads to GI permeability. After this intestinal disturbance, the mice exhibited adverse neurological behaviors that included anxiety, sensorimotor dysfunction, depression, and communication abnormalities. Afterward, these same mice were given a probiotic formula that reduced, if not corrected, their leaky gut and abnormal behaviors. Healthy human test subjects have also been treated with probiotic formulations, which also resulted in beneficial outcomes and improved cognitive function. These discoveries display the significant need for intestinal health and its role in physiological symptoms.

Like an overgrowth of specific intestinal bacteria, Candida albicans, a fungal yeast that lives largely in the digestive tract, is also of concern to an individual's health if excessive growth persists. For instance, a survey performed by the Autism Research Institute of over 25,000 parents reported that anti-fungal treatments were a highly effective means of improving their child's behavior. Candida infection plays a role in the immune system's ability to function properly, and like bacteria, causes a build-up of excessive toxic gases. While these gases are a natural waste product and part of the microbial metabolism, excessive gases produced by an overload of bad bacteria and fungi can cause brain fog and neurological disruption on a daily basis. All of this provides us a strong understanding that gut health is key to the overall improvement of physical and neurological health.

The Power of Bacteria and Fungus

The first, yet one of the most underestimated places to look regarding health is the human intestine. The GI system has over 1,000 different strains of intestinal bacteria. Some of these are good while others can be detrimental to health if left unchecked.

Ideally, the intestinal flora can operate in balance with one another, allowing for normal body function. However, when circumstances allow for an overgrowth of certain less desirable microorganisms, the result can be catastrophic and the symptoms can present themselves in multiple forms. This can mean chronic digestive problems, physical discomfort, irritability, speech delay, lack of attention, lethargy, autoimmune dysfunction, and many other outcomes for those affected.

Several studies reveal a connection between the type of bacteria in our gut and the resulting brain chemistry and behaviors associated with that bacteria. Some scientists believe that the bacteria found in our digestive system may help shape our brain structure and possibly influence our mood and behavior.

In one particular study, researchers analyzed two groups of mice that received fecal bacteria transplants from children. One group comprised children that had an autism spectrum disorder diagnosis, while the other group was made up of neurotypical children. The mice who received transplants from the ASD children exhibited autism-like behaviors such as reduced social interaction, diminished vocalization, and increased repetitive behaviors. Whereas the mice who received transplants from typical children did not. This lends insight that our intestine holds critical information regarding our health and daily function that begs serious consideration.

There are many factors that can contribute to negative intestinal overgrowth. Researchers have identified several possibilities. These include low acidity in the stomach, malnutrition, environmental stress, heavy metal toxicity, and excessive use of antibiotics. These circumstances can cause a hostile intestinal environment that may lead to bad bacterial overgrowth or candida.

Antibiotic therapy, by nature, causes a wide range of microbial changes. As we know, antibiotics work to kill off many bacteria in the intestine, including the beneficial ones. This then creates an environment in which pathogens can thrive and degrade intestinal mucosa leading to an inability to absorb nutrients. Let me add here that antibiotics are a life-saving scientific invention worthy of gratitude and praise. However, like many wonderful creations, antibiotics are often overprescribed for illnesses the body can manage on its own. For instance, parents of children with recurrent infections, particularly ear infections, should be wary of regular antibiotic use. Caretakers should be encouraged to look at diet first in such cases. Even the simple elimination of cow's milk has been found to clear up many recurring infections. And if antibiotics are a needed treatment, they should be given with a follow-up plan such as a probiotic post-program to help reinstate beneficial bacteria.

It is also important to note that if the intestinal balance is already compromised through environmental factors, a child's malnutrition may not be for lack of trying. Their body has become ill-equipped to absorb all the nutrients they receive due to existing intestinal permeability or leaky gut. By this point, a complete overhaul will be required to allow the body to rest, reset, and rebuild.

The Brain-Gut Connection

Direct communication occurs between the gut and brain through the vagus nerve. Therefore, if something is off within the intestine, the brain will receive that message and be subject to the state of the GI tract. Most of the time we will not notice these changes if we are consistently eating the same less-effective foods. Recurring mental or behavioral symptoms are then often chalked up to something else. However, this direct connection between the gut and brain means we have a great deal of power over how we or our children feel and respond to our environment.

Research has also displayed that what we eat can alter the composition and products of the gut flora. For instance, in another study individuals who consumed a high vegetable fiber-based diet, similar to that of early humans, had a different gut environment than those who consumed a typical Western diet high in low-quality fat, refined carbohydrates, and manufactured ingredients. Those who ate a more rural diet had balanced microbial diversity, allowing them to maximize energy intake and protect against inflammation and colonic diseases compared to those who typically ate a modern Western diet.

A negative chain of events occurs for those with GI distress. The pathogens in the intestinal tract feed off of undigested carbohydrates furthering the vitality of the bacteria and fungal overgrowth. At some point in the process, an injury takes place on the small intestine's surface, causing it to malfunction in its ability to digest incoming foods. From this, disaccharides, a specific family of sugars, are no longer digested properly and are left to linger in the small intestine. This then causes an all-you-can-eat buffet for bad bacteria, allowing them to multiply and create toxic byproducts within the intestine. Excessive mucus production then becomes a result of the inflammation and leads to diarrhea, bloating, and a host of physiological problems.

Inflammation affects healthy GI function and leads to a damaged intestinal lining that is unable to break down incoming carbohydrates. This damage then leads to leaky gut, a condition that allows harmful elements to seep into the bloodstream, furthering the digestive problems to more than just that. Now we're dealing with physiological symptoms that may include lethargy, anxiousness, depression, a poor ability to learn, and the list goes on.

Carbohydrate Reaction

Extensive research displays that individuals with autism, ADHD, and autoimmune dysfunction benefit from the elimination of certain foods from their diet. This includes specific carbohydrates, both complex and simple, as well as starch, refined sugars, artificial ingredients, casein, and gluten. By adhering to the Foods Four Thought Diet for a length of time, you will allow your child to eliminate their digestive ailments and reduce common behavioral and physical symptoms. As you heal the intestine and reduce inflammation, many health issues will be remedied. This includes adverse autoimmune responses, headaches, energy levels, and certain neurological challenges. Pairing these findings suggests a possibility that such a diet may successfully reduce the symptoms associated with these diagnoses—thus promoting a better quality of life for these children and their families.

In one study, a group of children diagnosed with Crohn's disease, which is a severe inflammation of the digestive organs, adhered to a selective carbohydrate diet similar to FFT. Every patient in that study experienced complete relief from their symptoms within a three-month intervention. Several other studies exist with similar results. This is relevant due to the common digestive inflammation that many of our unique children experience.

The Trouble with GFCF

The gluten-free, casein-free diet, also known as the GFCF diet, is a commonly suggested dietary intervention, particularly for children with autism. This is because specific proteins found within gluten and casein are often not tolerated by certain populations, including those with ASD and even ADHD. And while some do experience benefits from adhering to this diet alone, it usually falls short of what most hope to gain from it. Many of the packaged foods labeled "gluten-free" or "casein-free" remain full of, or simply are, ingredients that are difficult to digest within a compromised system. Foods containing starch, sugar, and complex grains will continue to feed a bad bacterial or fungal overgrowth that may already be present in the intestine.

The Autoimmune Link

Many children with autism and ADHD also experience autoimmune-related issues. These are noted as PANS/PANDAS, frequent thyroid dysfunction, psoriasis, compromised immunity, allergies, and other related symptoms. Not to mention Crohn's Disease and Colitis which are in and of themselves autoimmune diseases. Also important to note is that parents who have an autoimmune disorder are considerably more likely to have a child with any of the above diagnoses. With the prevalence of autoimmune disorders also on the rise, understanding this correlation is critical.

The Foods Four Thought Diet is beneficial for those with autoimmune disorders or simply those with sensitive systems, as it allows the intake of only easy to handle foods. This means you focus on nutrient-dense foods that the body can easily break down and use for energy. This allows inflammation to subside and the body to find a new rested level.

CHAPTER 4

WHAT IS FOODS FOUR THOUGHT?

Foods Four Thought is a way of eating that is built upon four primary food groups; fruit, vegetables, healthy fats, and lean proteins. We will also discuss the application of a vegan option without animal protein. The guidelines you will find here come together to create a way of eating that is effective and practical for children. Through the diet, you will set the stage for optimal health. This is done by eliminating foods that can do harm while amping up those that promote healing. And as mentioned before, it is ideal for all household members to take part as close to the diet as possible. This will ensure greater effectiveness and the ability to remain strict with the diet, providing optimal health for all family members.

To put it simply, the Foods Four Thought Diet is like pushing the reset button to your child's health. Imagine their inner function is a pipeline backed up with toxic sludge. To get things running properly again, we must clear out the sludge, clean the pipes, patch the holes, and get it running smoothly once again. It can then be used properly forever afterward by putting the correct fuel in and letting it filter out—never allowing it to build up to that problematic mess it once was.

Many foods are deemed healthy because of their vitamin or mineral content, yet they negatively impact our children with unique needs who are, at present, unable to digest them properly. The FFT Diet eliminates these problematic foods for an extension of time. This allows the body to recover and inflammation to subside. Many of these foods can, however, be reintroduced in later stages of the diet as we will discuss later on. You may question if food really is a problematic trigger for your child. However, you might not recognize that a particular food is a culprit to challenging physical symptoms or behaviors because it is eaten more or less daily. If this is the case, certain symptoms would appear as expected or the norm. But eliminate these foods, and the difference their absence makes will amaze you.

One goal of the diet is to create a reasonably sustainable way of eating so that your child can feel and function their absolute best possible. Through the diet, you will have the opportunity to change how you think about food. This will happen as you witness your and your child's improved daytime energy, sleep patterns, mental clarity, alleviation from digestive dysfunction, acne, allergies, ear infections, hives, and other challenges improve.

How the Diet Works

It's crucial to understand and believe the *why's* behind the FFT Diet's ability to heal, thus we discussed the research in chapter three. Having a conviction that sticking to the protocol will work in time will provide you the mental, emotional, and physical strength to continue your journey through the diet, and witness the power of nutrition. Thus, we will revisit certain information and research discussed previously to understand the need and benefits of the Foods Four Thought Diet.

Many of our children with unique needs have low carbohydrate digestive enzyme activity. This means they are not equipped to utilize incoming carbohydrates effectively. Therefore, it is imperative to supply them with a diet that their body can manage. Further, the diet works to starve off the bad bacteria and fungal overgrowth, which typically feed off of undigested carbohydrates within the intestine. As you restore microbial balance in the gut, healing of intestinal permeability can begin. This healing then provides a reduction of physical and behavioral problems.

The Foods Four Thought Diet involves removing all simple and complex carbohydrates, starches, processed foods, and sugars —except for those found in honey and fruit. This means that grains and starchy vegetables such as potatoes and corn will also be eliminated to allow for optimal healing.

Foods permitted on this diet are lean meats such as poultry, eggs, and fish, nuts, seeds, and non-starchy vegetables. Fruit and honey are also permitted because of how they break down in the body, meaning these are foods that will not feed existing bacteria or fungal overgrowth. Other foods such as certain beans can be carefully added during the later phases of the diet. We will discuss the process of doing this in an upcoming chapter.

The FFT Diet is a means of eating which nourishes the body while starving off intestinal bacteria or candida that causes various ailments and behavioral disruptions. We will use the diet as a catalyst for resolving these digestive issues. If your child does not appear to have intestinal dysfunction, the diet is still beneficial for them. This is because they are eating low-stress foods with maximum nutrition. And while the diet is intended to be temporary, many strive to make it a lifestyle because of the ease in which the body can utilize nutrients within the four food pillars.

How Long Does the Diet Take to Work?

I highly recommend that your child is 100% compliant with the rules of the diet for at least two months before slowly adding in any other food groups. After two months, you can slowly but surely experiment with one new food at a time. During this period, you may also discover food intolerances that you did not realize were present prior to the dietary elimination.

This prospectively short amount of time will allow you to see if diet modification is what your child needs. If you do not see improvement within the first two months then there is likely something else at play and further discovery will need to be made. However, this short timeline means you must be strictly adherent. Improvements cannot be made, and you cannot accurately know if the diet is working if the child is still having occasional treats or non-approved foods. This is because each little bit of sugar means a small refeed for the pathogens and thus a step backward in the healing process.

If within these first two months you are seeing improvements in either digestion, health, comfort, behaviors, or learning, then keep going! This diet is what your child's body is needing and healing is underway. But this process takes time. If you end too early, you will halt improvement and may see regression. As I mentioned before, we remained on the diet for four years. Not because it was necessary, but because it was so successful and I was terrified to stray. Plus, we had learned how to make eating this way work within our lifestyle. My suggestion is to remain in Phase One, eating FFT approved foods for as long as you're reasonably willing and able. Two months is the minimum and twelve months is ideal. Afterward, you can very slowly experiment with reintroducing whole foods such as quinoa and other non-gluten grains or beans.

Journal Everything

As you move through the diet, it will be imperative to keep a journal. In this, you will record what foods your child eats each day and any associated behaviors. Writing information down is an effective way to track what foods your child may respond to positively or negatively. This is also an opportunity to document new improvements. These will help you draw inspiration on harder days. So invest in a journal of your preference that is specifically intended for your Foods Four Thought journey. I have listed one that is particularly great on the Products page of the Foods Four Thought website, www.foodsfourthought.com/products. Here you will also find a children's food journal to add a layer of involvement and learning, which is recommended.

My Child Doesn't Have GI Problems. Will the Diet Still Help?

While I'd love to give a resounding "Yes! The diet is everything you've been searching for" to everyone who makes the changes, there can be no guarantee. All I can testify is the incredible impact it had in our own lives, many of the children I've worked with, and the data that supports why this diet works for so many. If your child is among the percentage of children who do not have digestive problems, there is still a significant probability that the diet will promote improved physical symptoms, behaviors, and learning ability. The foods on this diet are absolutely packed with nutrients that the brain and body need. So yes, the FFT Diet holds power for you too. And there's only one way to know if it will work for sure. Take the plunge and give it a solid go for two prospectively short months.

Foods Four Thought Diet

CHAPTER 5

ALL ABOUT FOOD

Now we'll thoroughly discuss what foods are and are not permitted while on the diet. The information here will provide you with the tools you need to make good decisions and take control of your and your child's health.

What Not to Eat and Why

As mentioned before, many of the foods in this section are considered "nutritious" because of either their high fiber content or value in certain vitamins or minerals. However, if these healthy foods are intolerable to the consumer, for whatever reason, they are useless and even damaging. So you can better understand what foods to omit over these next few months, I have broken them down for you here. Digest the information completely. The following foods will prevent healing. They may not have to be off-limits forever, but as for the time being, do not allow them within your child's diet.

Whole Grains — For the next few months, avoid all grains and grain seeds. This includes wheat, rice, oats, quinoa, corn, buckwheat, barley, rye, semolina, and several others. Whole grains can definitely contain a great deal of health-promoting benefits, but for those who are not currently equipped to handle them, they can cause an excess of inflammation. This then manifests itself in behavioral, emotional, and physical ways. What's more is that whole grains contain phytic acid. This substance binds to and inhibits proper digestion of certain minerals such as calcium, magnesium, iron, and zinc. This makes the nutrients partially unavailable for absorption despite the food's actual content. Because of this process grains are nutrient-poor when compared to fruits and vegetables.

Legumes — This includes beans, peas, lentils, soy, and peanuts. These foods have similar problems as grains as they also contain phytic acid. This too makes them nutrient-poor when compared to eating fruit and vegetables. If you include legumes after you have obtained complete intestinal healing, make a habit of preparing these foods from home instead of purchasing them pre-canned from the store. This will allow you to properly soak, rinse, and cook them—something most manufacturers do not take the time to do. Soaking your legumes reduces their levels of phytic acid, making them more nutritious. Further, this can help dissolve their outer shell, which will help them digest more appropriately without causing digestive problems.

Soy — Soybeans are part of the legume family, but deserve a special mention because of their problematic nature. You will need to pass on any product containing soy while implementing the Foods Four Thought Diet and will want to avoid it as much as possible forever after. The reason is that soy is now commonly over-processed to the point of being intolerable to the body. Most soy products you find on the back of food labels are a far cry from the purely fermented soybeans originally grown in ancient Asia. Soy products also contain phytoestrogen compounds, which may be linked to an increased susceptibility to several types of cancers within specific populations. Soy, even pure forms such as tofu or tempeh, block mineral absorption due to phytate. This is the last thing your nutrient-deficient child needs, thus, I heartily recommend eradicating soy for your child undergoing the healing process. So, instead of eating tofu, opt for lean meat, or strictly vegetable dishes. And in sauces, use coconut aminos over soy sauce. These are delicious and not too difficult to find anymore.

Peanuts — These are also part of the legume family, but because of their high availability and tasty allure, we'll discuss them specifically. Peanuts are high in lectins, which are resistant to digestion. They also contain specific proteins that promote significant inflammation once they cross into the bloodstream. Consider the prevalence of peanut allergies and how dangerous they can be. Instead of peanuts, you can try a range of tree nuts and seeds as snacks, and nut or seed butter instead of traditional peanut butter.

Artificial Sweeteners — These can promote overall poor body function and discourage the eradication of pathogens in the intestine. Their chemical structures will most often cause continued feeding for the bacteria or fungus. These will also range in their level of safety. Some are semi-natural, having been modified and processed in a lab. While others really have no business being available to the public and have actually been banned in certain countries.

Alcohol — Outside of being a recreational drink, alcohol can be found in flavor extracts such as vanilla and almond extract. This substance is often broken down in the system as sugar and is not allowed while on the diet. If you are seriously considering taking this venture with your child, which is highly recommended, you will want to give up all alcohol consumption. It contains no actual nutrition and can affect the integrity of the intestinal lining, thus contributing to inflammatory problems.

Dairy — This includes all forms of animal milk, cheese, and yogurt. Dairy can cause a harmful immune response in many individuals, sometimes without us knowing. This is because of its inflammatory proteins. Lactose is a carbohydrate that is found in milk. When this carbohydrate binds with the protein in milk an inflammatory response is triggered. Casein, a dairy protein, can also lead to inflammation and is associated with an increased risk of autoimmune disease. Last, immune factors within milk protein can react with our immune system, leading to greater severity of allergies, infections, and acne.

There are many excellent substitutions for traditional milk, butter, and yogurt. Consider coconut milk and oil or almond milk. It's challenging to find a proper substitution for cheese, so just plan on omitting all things cheesy for now.

Ghee may be an exception to this rule regarding dairy. Ghee is prepared in a way that causes traceable levels of lactose and casein to be eliminated. It also has other health benefits such as probiotics, anticarcinogenic properties, and the ability to carry critical fat-soluble vitamins such as A, D, E, and K.

When it is time to reintroduce dairy, consider starting with goat products. These contain less lactose, thus are better tolerated. Goat dairy products have a breathy quality in their flavor, but it's not bad, and something you and your child could get used to.

High Glutamate Foods — Glutamate occurs naturally within the body and in many foods. However, an excess of this amino acid can contribute to numerous problems, particularly within the brain. These can include headache, anxiety, depression, and mood swings. Foods high in glutamate have largely already been discussed and include MSG, many artificial sweeteners, and soy products. Others to be wary of include tomatoes, mushrooms, peas, parmesan cheese, processed meat, yeast, and cows milk. These foods will be eliminated during Phase One and should be carefully assessed if reintroduced later as you watch for aversive reactions.

There is good to be found in nearly all whole food grown from the ground or free-roaming. However, you must be able to differentiate if something is good, better, or best. This is because some "good" foods may cause harm due to an individual's present intolerance. For instance, we understand that grains and beans provide fiber and that dairy has calcium. However, there isn't a nutrient, vitamin, mineral, or phytonutrient that you can't get from eating an array of fruits, vegetables, healthy fats, and lean proteins. And most foods found within these groups will not contribute to the inflammatory downsides that otherwise come from grains that dilute vital nutrient uptake or dairy that promotes excessive mucus creation.

It is important to remember that many of the current off-limits foods can be successfully reintroduced in their own time and eaten sparingly. This can be done successfully if the four food pillars continue to make up the bulk of the diet now and forever after.

The prohibited foods listed previously will need to be eliminated to understand how optimal your child's functioning can be. Thus, you will avoid them at all costs for the next several months while you allow your child's body to rebalance and find a new ideal. This means no nibbles, tastes, or sips. Even small bites can set the body backward in its healing path. Give the body a chance to restore its natural balance. Allow it to heal and recover, and allow your family an opportunity to change and create new positive habits and methods of eating.

Pay close attention to everything. See what changes as you take daily notes and write in your child's diet and health journal. In a couple of months, you will reintroduce many previously eliminated foods one at a time. Then, with systematic caution, you can test if or how certain foods are sending your child's system off balance.

In this promising short time, you will know what doctors or other caretakers could not figure out. You can identify what the ideal diet looks like for your child, and perhaps for you as well. You will know the foods that feel the most sustainable, wholesome, and satisfying. This will be the diet that keeps your child healthy and feeling their best. In time, they will be able to occasionally have foods that do not allow optimal function, because that is life. There will always be a party or a holiday dinner. Planning around these will be a challenge for the first little while, but it will be necessary. However, in the future, your child can eat the foods prepared by friends or family without the negative reactions, or at the very least, you will know what the repercussions may be and how to bounce back to a healthy diet after the event.

What You Can Eat

Meet our heroes. The four food groups that will promote the best, most effective nutrients without the physical or neurological stress that the previous foods are inclined to create. These can be eaten without limitation unless an allergy exists to a specific food within any of these groups. Essentially, what is allowed or not allowed to be eaten is largely based on the food's chemical structure. If it has a complex structure and can ferment while in the digestive tract, it cannot be eaten. Thus comes the allowance of almost all vegetables, fruit, honey, nuts, seeds, natural oils, and lean organic animal protein. These foods allow for undisrupted digestion and improved nourishment.

Vegetables — These are allowed throughout the course of the diet, except for those that are higher in starch. This means that potatoes, parsnips, cassava, corn, and even green peas will need to be avoided while on the diet. Starches break down within the body similar to sugar. They are all nutritious in their own right but won't help facilitate rapid healing of the intestinal tract, therefore will need to be eliminated during Phase One.

Also, worthy of mention is the consumption of cruciferous vegetables. These are those lovely gassy veggies such as cabbage, broccoli, Brussels sprouts, and cauliflower. I suggest minimizing these for the first month, eating them sparingly. These will not feed the harmful bacteria that we are trying to kill off but can promote gas and discomfort, especially within a poorly performing digestive system.

Also, for the first couple of weeks, you will want to cook as much food as you can before consumption, especially if diarrhea was severe prior to the diet. Cooking food first can help with digestion. Raw fruit and vegetables have a higher nutrient profile, but right now we are focused on getting the child to eat in the first place and helping them to be as comfortable throughout the day as possible. You can add raw fruits or vegetables daily at your discretion—just be sure to keep notes in your journal if you do.

An excellent way to get your kids to eat more vegetables is to make soup, and if they are sensory sensitive, you can make pureed soups with lots of lovely spices. You will find several pureed soup recipes later in the book that are delicious and simple to make. What I also love about pureed soup is you can make it in large batches and freeze it for future use.

Herbs and spices can be used freely. If you are buying a packaged seasoning blend, be sure to check for any unnatural fillers. These are often incorporated to reduce clumping while in storage. As always, try to use the freshest ingredients possible.

Fruit — Most fruit can be eaten without problems. Some children will continue to experience diarrhea if too much fruit is consumed, thus, watch for this and as a general rule allow a small portion of fruit as a dessert after a meal or part of a small snack. For example, some sliced peaches after dinner will satisfy a sweet tooth. Bananas will require the most caution before eating. It will be important to make sure the bananas are plenty ripe with a fair amount of brown spots and no green stems. Under-ripe bananas digest similar to starch, which you do not want. Plantains also are too starchy to be allowed within the first stage of the diet.

Smoothies are a great way to get kids, or adults for that matter, to eat fruit and vegetables. Smoothies are also excellent because they are pureed, thus easier to digest even if they are not cooked.

I will add that I suggest sticking to fruit with a lower glycemic index profile within the first two weeks, then add sweeter ones such as bananas and pineapples, later on, one at a time. Elimination of harmful pathogens is often most successful and rapid when you can keep anything sweet to a minimum. In chapter eleven you will find a chart that displays preferred low GI fruits compared to higher GI fruits.

Fats — Nuts, seeds, and plant oils are a great way to get quality calories and fats into the diet. Using healthy oils such as coconut oil, avocado oil, and olive oil is freely permitted and even encouraged. More often than not, picky eaters are underweight, therefore including these high-quality fats will ensure they are getting the caloric energy they need to have a successful day. Even if your child is not underweight, they will still benefit from consuming plenty of these high-quality foods. These natural oils are also health-promoting for brain and cardiac health, so include them where you can. I suggest diversifying your use of oils to get the most out of their individual benefits as much as possible. This might look like putting coconut oil in your smoothies for added flavor and energy, cooking with avocado oil, and using olive oil in your salad dressings. There are some incredible salad dressing recipes later in this book, and while your child may not be up for eating salads anytime soon, you can still experiment and perhaps you or another member of your household can enjoy them if your child won't right away. It took my son several months before he would tolerate a salad because of their varied texture, but now they are amongst his top favorite meals. Also, do your best to avoid canola oil, safflower oil, and soybean oil. These oils are highly over-processed and are frequently genetically modified.

As for nuts and seeds, these are a great snack to have available and will definitely satiate hunger pains. However, these foods will need to be consumed in moderation. Overconsumption of nuts and seeds will often cause cramping or constipation, especially within a sensitive digestive tract. Therefore, you will see coconut flour in the baked goods recipes later in the book as opposed to almond flour. This allows room for nuts, seeds, and their butters to be eaten without overdoing them in total. You can certainly use almond flour for baking, but you may run into digestive problems if nuts are eaten elsewhere within the day. If you are weary of nuts being a problematic food for your child, introduce only one type of nut or seed at a time. Wait four days between trying another to check for tolerance.

Protein — Lean meats are also an important way to get daily nutrients and can make up a fair portion of the diet. Meats to include are fish, poultry, and eggs—so long as eggs are not an allergen for the individual. Animal protein does not perpetuate inflammation thus is allowed on the diet. It is important to know that meat definitely has its ranks regarding what can optimize digestion and bodily function.

Fish is the most acceptable, particularly wild-caught Alaskan salmon and cod. It is imperative that you absolutely avoid any fish that contains tripolyphosphate. It should be listed on the ingredients label and is commonly found in frozen, store-bought fish. This is a suspected neurotoxic preservative and is frequently used when fish is caught far across the globe and must be shipped long distances. This preservative has been linked to several harmful side effects including malabsorption and inflammation within the intestine, which is definitely the last thing we need right now.

Poultry is also acceptable but in moderate quantities. You should seek out farmers that raise organic, free-range poultry, and whom you can speak with if possible. Chickens or turkeys that are fed a vegetarian diet is not good enough. Nowadays the common poultry farming method is to give the animals gluten, soy, or corn feed. This can pass into the animal's tissues, causing them to become saturated with these problematic foods. This same rule goes for eggs. If you cannot find a local farmer who raises true free-range, soy-free chickens or wild turkeys, your nearest health food store should have what you're looking for. If you cannot find any local stores or farmers that raise their birds using natural pasture-raised methods, then omit poultry or eat it sparingly—being sure to take notes on any adverse reactions.

As for pork, beef, and other red meat, I recommend these be avoided altogether. They are more difficult to digest compared to other sources of animal protein, and have been significantly linked to high blood pressure and type 2 diabetes. Plus, they are generally no longer a sustainable food source considering the overall current population. These animals, namely cows and pigs, take up far too much farmland, create an excess of waste products, and contribute considerably to greenhouse gasses. While these latter reasons are not directly diet-related, they are still of the utmost importance to human and global health.

If you are vegan or want to consume a high plant-based diet, this is no problem. Your child will definitely be able to benefit from the vast array of other foods available on this diet.

Honey and Coconut Sugar — These are the only allowed natural sweeteners. Because of their simple chemical structure, they can break down with ease without feeding pathogens. They are a great addition to sweet treats, and you will see them repeatedly within the recipes. Coconut syrup and date sugar are also acceptable substitutes. Just be sure when you purchase these from the store they are labeled organic and do not contain added ingredients. Maple and agave syrup are not allowed while on the diet because of their more complex sugar bond. Stevia is also not recommended while in Phase One as it can cause bloating and discomfort in some. You might consider adding it later on.

As you see, there are a lot of amazing food options that your child can still enjoy. Now, I will not tell you it's easy because it's not. Number one, you are trying to get a child to eat what you tell them. This is always a chore, no matter the challenges of the child. And number two, this is a child who may have intensely set rules around what they want to eat and why. But, it can be done with positive energy, communication, and planning. Just be sure that everything you buy is as close to natural as possible. Meaning it is labeled non-GMO, organic, or is purchased from a reputable local farmer. Sticking to these foods will be the key to finding your child's best level of health at this time in their life.

Over the years of talking with caregivers who are considering making dietary changes for their child, I have come in contact with many who tell me that their child would rather starve. I get it, you have a super picky eater. But in reality, the number of children who are literally willing to starve is few. There are very rare cases in which a child will completely forsake their instinctual need to survive. Your child is more than likely equipped to completely adhere to the food outlined here. We'll talk more about proceeding safely and confidently in an upcoming chapter.

Introducing Foods Later

Home-prepared beans and legumes are a great addition to the diet in later phases, as they can be a good source of plant-based protein, folate, and potassium, just to name a few critical nutrients. Non-gluten grains such as oats and rice are also a nice addition if tolerated later on as they can add meal diversity and varied nutrients.

As you now know, you will be able to slowly and strategically introduce foods outside of these four pillars once your child has achieved intestinal balance. We will get specific on this process and how this can be achieved in chapter eight.

Supplements

You've likely done a fair amount of research and dabbling in supplements already. Most of our kids with unique needs are inclined to be nutrient deficient for several reasons, particularly in specific vitamins and minerals. So, let's take some time to discuss supplementation as it will be of some importance moving forward.

Multivitamin — Taking a multivitamin and mineral supplement is recommended but unnecessary if the child has gained a broad range of food that they will eat. Anyone who has had prolonged intestinal disruption is likely malnourished and thus will benefit from additional micronutrient nourishment. However, you must check the labels closely. It's difficult, if not impossible, to find kids vitamins that don't contain ingredients that will feed existing pathogens. This commonly includes added sweeteners, fillers, or thickeners. You can check with the Allowed and Non-Permitted list of ingredients in chapter eleven to see if the supplements you have on hand make the cut.

Ultimately, my rule of thumb is to allow the child a multivitamin if they are willing and able to swallow them in pill form or you can mix them into their food. Otherwise, if they will only take a liquid, gummy, or chewable vitamin, I suggest holding off for the first two months or longer. The truth is, if your child is slowly continuing to broaden their diet and the list of foods they are willing to eat is growing, this should be adequate for now. The four permitted food groups contain highly nutritious foods, and if eaten in a balanced manner they should be enough for your child. Suppose however, they have a medical condition or are following physicians' orders. In that case, it is a whole different matter and I certainly won't suggest that they stop taking something that is prescribed or heavily advocated by your child's doctor.

Probiotics — These are also important in healing and will further promote good bacteria in the intestine and expedite the recovery of the gut and balanced flora. A significant amount of study has been done to validate the success of including probiotics as a daily supplement, as has been mentioned in previous chapters. Because our intestine works best when there is a relative balance of good bacteria, I suggest purchasing three different probiotic formulas and rotating them. Alternatively, you can order one complete formula that has a relatively balanced ratio of bacterial strains. You can view recommendations in the Additional Resources section or check out the Products page on the Foods Four Thought website. As mentioned before, probiotics are a powerful tool for health and should be part of any daily routine whether you are ill or not. However, the most common side effect of probiotics, especially within a sensitive system, is diarrhea. This can cause obvious problems or discomfort, thus consider introducing a new probiotic on a day when you and your child will be home. Also, introduce only a small amount and move upward from there toward the suggested dose.

You can also receive a great deal of probiotic benefits by eating fermented foods. However, I find these are typically difficult to get children to eat due to their unique taste, so I won't go further on that here, but there are plenty of good resources at the library and through the internet on fermented foods. Lastly, you can also make coconut yogurt and kefir using a non-dairy starter. It's a bit of work, but well worth it for some.

Fish Oil — The benefits of high-quality fish oil are many. It is useful to health throughout the lifespan, from the womb, and into old age. Countless studies display its health-promoting benefits. Regarding our unique kids and their current needs, it has been shown to be an aid to reducing hyperactivity, anxiety, improve immune function, academic performance, mood, and continued neurodevelopmental growth.

Like with anything, you will want to be sure to get high-quality fish oil that is not diluted with other filler oils such as safflower oil or soybean oil. Also, just like the fish your family will be eating, be sure you are getting fish oil from wild-caught, and preferably Alaskan fish.

When beginning any supplement, the rule is to take it four days in a row, provided it does not cause concern right away. During this time, never introduce anything else new. That way, if there are beneficial or adverse effects, you will know which supplement to credit. As always, journal these results.

Ultimately, as the Greek philosopher, Hippocrates said, "Let food be thy medicine, and medicine be thy food." We can take supplements to give us a leg up, but nothing can come close to the healing benefits of a wholesome and complete diet that is tailored to a person's specific needs.

Your action step now is to check any existing supplements your child may be taking. Make sure there are no non-preferred ingredients. If a supplement does not align with the diet, look for a different one that will. Alternatively, you can just lay off of them for a bit if you are comfortable doing so. As always, you are welcome to discuss all things with your child's primary health care provider or alternative medicine specialist.

Foods Four Thought vs. Other Diets

The wheel has not been reinvented here with the FFT Diet. There are many incredible diets out there that do a fantastic job of healing the body. What sets the elements within this book apart is that it has kept our children's sensory sensitivities in mind, including their inclined inability to metabolize certain foods, plus your busy schedule. Many elimination diets such as SCD, GAPS, AIP, or paleo are wonderful and significantly better than following the current Western diet, or even the approved food pyramid. Each of these distinguished diets shares similarities and also carries relative differences, primarily in their introduction phases, if they have one at all. Each diet's details can be easily researched, so we won't go into them here.

What makes Foods Four Thought ideal for your family is the ease of the menu, shopping, meal prep, and kid-friendly recipes. There is also no major introductory process and you can eat fruit while on the diet, something other diets shy away from. Last, the upcoming communication tools will help get your child involved with the process of eating healthy.

So now, please take a moment and look over the approved four food groups once more, and skim through the full list of foods that are and are not permitted in chapter eleven. You will use this as an important reference, especially while checking labels at the grocery store. This list is highly comprehensive, so if an item is not on the list, then assume it's not approved because of its chemical structure and difficulty to digest.

CHAPTER 6

COMMUNICATION

One of the most essential elements of this diet and a vital key to its success is communication. This means presenting basic information about the new diet with your child, any household members, and people who are part of their daily life and who will need to know your current restrictions around food. If your child struggles with communication, this is okay. As I mentioned before, my son was non-verbal when we implemented dietary changes, and most of the families I've worked with also had non-verbal children. For this reason, we will use the power of physical visuals to communicate the changes. The tools you will find here and in upcoming chapters will serve you well and help minimize trial and error.

Interactive Menu

When my son started the diet, I created a visual chart of the things he could eat and divided them into food groups. This helped him know the changes that were going to be made. It was also something I could easily get out whenever he needed a reminder and was helpful when he got frustrated that previous favorites were not available.

The visual chart consisted of a blank and laminated menu page and little laminated square picture tiles with Velcro on the back. These displayed various allowed foods on each one. From this, he could pick and stick the foods he wanted at different points in the day. It was a great tool because it got him directly involved in the process, and because there was only one picture tile of each food, this forced him to think outside of his box and pick some new foods to try. He didn't always eat these new foods, but with time and exposure, he came around. Your child will also give way to broadening their diet if you are consistently trying. It's not a perfect process, so only offer small amounts of each new food. In this way, you will minimize your frustration and reduce waste. The interactive menu was such a success and my son enjoyed it, thus I have made it easily available on the website at www.foodsfourthought.com/kids-menu. You can print this out for your child and allow them to engage in choosing their food. I suggest laminating the board and tiles for the sake of durability.

If you are trying to get an older child or teen on board, these visuals may not be necessary. Alternatively, you can also adapt them and tailor their use to your specific child and their needs or interests. Including them and allowing your child as much freedom as you can possibly provide is so important in this and any process. You don't need to be a tyrant to get this diet to work. In fact, it can't work with extreme force. This process should be approached with calm and unity as much as is possible.

Interactive Health Checklist

Another great way to approach communication about this diet is to discuss what benefits the child may experience if they adhere to it for the next while. This will be most successful for older children or those without a significant communication barrier. Is there something that particularly troubles them? Do they hate their stomachaches or earaches? Do they want to focus better during the day? If they are teens or pre-teens, do they want their acne to clear up? Helping them recognize that this diet may help them with these troubles is also a potentially powerful tool to get them on board and electively adhering to the diet. You can download this interactive health checklist if you feel it will be helpful at www.foodsfourthought.com/kids-checklist. Once printed out, they can check off the items relevant to them.

Interactive Calendar Goal

I also recommend having a calendar available on which your child can mark if they had a successful day of eating. Depending on the child you can decide how far out to set a prize date. Younger children will typically only be able to wait a maximum of one week. Older children could potentially make it two weeks or even one month if the prize is incentivizing enough. After they have been one hundred percent with the diet for the decided amount of time, you can celebrate by going bowling or buying a new Lego set, whatever appeals to them personally. A little bribery can go a long way and is a powerful tool. At no point however, should you make this a food-related prize. You may find that even after two months you want to continue strict adherence to the diet, thus, you would not want to set a date for a pizza party. Additionally, pairing food as a reward can lead to a counterproductive way of thinking about food. Once the prize is won, set a new date and continue working towards that. You can get a special calendar that is in line with your child's interests or print one that I created for you at www.foodsfourthought.com/kids-calendar.

Ultimately, communication in whatever way your child can receive and reciprocate it, will be imperative to the diet's success. You will also need to communicate your dietary plans for your child with teachers, caretakers, grandparents, and other household members. This can be harder than it should be, just as fair warning. I've talked with many parents who were trying to get their child's diet on the right track only to run into their greatest obstacle being someone who should have been supportive. However, thankfully this is not always the case. You may be gifted with understanding, accepting, and generally easy-going people in your life. But if not, it's okay. We'll talk more about how to handle this in an upcoming chapter.

For now, take some time to digest and look through the website pages mentioned. Print off and prepare whichever ones you believe are most appropriate for your child. Have them ready to use as you start a dialogue to help your child understand what the diet will look like and why you believe it is crucial for them.

CHAPTER 7

READY TO BEGIN

Setting a Start Date

Let's now explore the actions of officially getting started. First, set a start date. Allow enough time to do your food prep, clear your cupboards of non-approved foods, talk to anyone who needs to be informed about your child's new dietary needs, and get your child prepared for the changes ahead.

When considering a start date, I suggest just going for it. Set it sometime within the next two weeks. Don't wait for a birthday party, holiday, or vacation to pass unless these are approaching within the next week. There will always be an event that makes sticking to the diet challenging. Don't plan around these. We'll discuss how to be successful despite such circumstances. So, decide which day of the week is best for food prep, and begin the diet the day after that.

Clear Your Cupboards

Before starting the diet, I highly suggest clearing out your fridge and cupboards of any problematic foods. If you have a significant other resistant to giving up their own preferred foods, remind them of what is at stake and ask for their support as you endeavor in this process and road to healing. Hopefully, that does the trick and your loved one hops on board. However, if they are unwilling to be supportive in this regard, you will expressly require them to keep their stash in a separate location out of sight and out of the kitchen. If it's chips or cookies, they can keep these in a bedroom or office drawer. If it's something that requires refrigeration, purchase a mini-fridge—it will be worth the small investment to keep the kitchen clean and clear. I also strongly suggest that you implore this person to keep their snacking and fast food runs private. Otherwise, it could tempt those in the home who are practicing the diet. It really will be imperative to keep the kitchen a safe space for healthy eats.

Setting a start date should give you enough time to eat any non-approved foods already in your kitchen if you prefer not to waste the money spent on them. If you're unable to make your way through these foods before your start date, consider donating any unopened items to a local shelter and dumping what has not yet been finished in the garbage.

Going Shopping

Let's start this section with a challenge. I encourage you to commit at this moment to stop buying non-approved items from the grocery store. For some, this may seem obvious, while others still may feel pressure to continue buying favorite boxed or bagged foods for certain household members. If the latter is you, this challenge may be difficult to wrap your head around. However, putting your foot down and insisting that everyone in the home eat the healthy food that you will buy and prepare is heavily encouraged. You will surely be met with resistance. If other household members dislike this new rule and are unwilling to abide by it, then let them know that they will have to pick up any non-approved items and eat them privately. If they cannot drive due to age, disability, or accessibility, then tough cookies. They will ride out this diet with everyone else. Drawing clear lines for everyone will significantly improve your ability to make this diet a success and better ensure you and your child get the most out of this healing process.

While on the diet, you will avoid ninety percent of what you will find on the interior isles of the supermarket. The days of buying cereal, crackers, and freezer meals are behind you. Instead, stock up on the items listed from the shopping list and anything else from the permitted list of foods you feel you or your child will enjoy eating. It's also highly encouraged that your child helps you at the grocery store. Get them to pick out the fruit or veggies that look interesting to them or that they might be willing to try. This will be an excellent experience for them on multiple levels. This does mean more work for you in monitoring them as they take part in the grocery shopping, but it's worth the extra effort.

Also, read every label of every bottle, box, or bag before placing it in your cart. Pre-packaged foods are riddled with ingredients that will stifle intestinal healing. The most common culprits in foods that should be healthy but are ruined by junk ingredients are sugar and soy. Sugar can also be in anything that states "from concentrate", so steer clear of foods with that statement unless the package expressly states "no sugar". Watch for other ingredients that we've discussed that are not approved while on the diet. When in doubt, check the Allowed and Non-permitted list provided in chapter eleven. However, it is best to prepare foods from scratch. This way, you can fully ensure your child is getting only whole foods and you know exactly what is in them.

It is a common misconception that eating healthy food costs significantly more money. And while that idea could have merit if paired up against certain factors, one study done by Harvard revealed that it costs only $1.50 more per day, per person to eat healthily. That's it. You could probably go and find six quarters under your couch cushions right now. You may think, *Well, that's $45 per month for each of us*. But if you consider averted therapy, hospital, or medication costs for any single person in your household, that $45 is nothing. So, in the grand scheme of things, even for a home of four people, $180 is insignificant compared to a better quality of life for the family.

The Meal Plan

As promised, you will find a sample 1-week meal plan in chapter eleven. This plan is one week of food for four people. A lot of the main meals here are soups that are meant to be pureed. I have created it this way understanding that a lot of our kids have sensory issues with food, therefore chewing or experiencing an array of textures all at once is aversive. Pureed soup and smoothies have the highest rate of success. However, if you feel your child can handle more than this, you can look through the Foods Four Thought website under Recipes for a greater variety of delicious meals.

Take a look at the meal plan. If it checks out for you, then proceed with the shopping list and buy the items listed there if you don't have them already. The shopping list directly coincides with the meal plan. Thus, if you omit a recipe from the meal plan, you will want to make necessary changes to the shopping list. I suggest doing much of your grocery shopping at a bulk store such as Costco or Sam's Club. These stores are generally good about keeping organic foods on hand at a reduced price. For other items, try to find a health food store near you. Buying items at a health food store does not guarantee that it will be appropriate for the diet, so continue to check labels if something catches your eye.

Meal Prep

If you don't meal prep already, you may find that it can be a lifesaver in the world of a busy and weary parent. It's a whole mess of work upfront but pays off big time throughout the week. Having fruit already cut up, breakfast muffins ready to go in the morning, or soup frozen and prepared to thaw after a long day will support greater opportunity for success. It will also ensure that you don't give in to a fast and easy but non-approved snack when you're in a rush or too exhausted to do much more than put something on a plate.

If possible, try making your shopping and meal prep all part of the same day. It helps the week feel less hectic if you're able to get related jobs done at similar times. So, go shopping in the morning, put on a movie for your kids when you get home, and meal prep to your favorite audiobook that same afternoon. If you're not able to grocery shop until evening, then just meal prep in your next available two to three hours, or find a schedule that allows you to get these two crucial tasks done within a similar part of your week.

Try to make sure you have nothing too pressing that evening because you will be tired. Make space on these days for some quality time alone or adequate relaxation—whatever that looks like for you.

If meal prepping is new to you, it's the process of chunking all of your cooking or meal preparation into one or two parts of the week as opposed to every day. This means you will spend this day dicing veggies, seasoning meat, baking muffins, and pureeing dressing to last you the week. It's a lot of work but it really pays off. If feasible, I suggest setting aside at least two hours on two different days to keep items as fresh as possible.

Your grocery list and 1-week meal plan are based on an ovo-vegetarian diet. If you are not vegetarian, then feel free to add some baked salmon or chicken on the side of your dinners. You can find wonderful and easy meat recipes on the website. If you are vegan, you will want to swap out the honey for coconut nectar on some meals. The baked goods will also need to be substituted for something else, as they contain eggs. You can again refer to the website for more vegan options.

Take a look at the meal plan and make any adjustments you feel will be needed for your family. You can plan on repeating this meal plan each week, or if you're feeling adventurous, you can find many recipes on the website. Other trusted recipe outlets are listed in the Additional Resources section as well. Just be sure to watch for needed adjustments if the recipes do not come from this book or the Foods Four Thought website. For instance, if something calls for butter, you now know to substitute for coconut oil. If a recipe calls for soy sauce, you can use coconut aminos, and so on. I've included a basic substitution chart to help with this in chapter eleven. Also, if you make any changes to the 1-week meal plan, be sure to make a thorough list of needed grocery items based on your week's recipes and desired snacks before you go shopping, so you are not left wanting for anything.

Again, I strongly suggest getting your family involved in the diet as much as possible. This ensures that the dietary changes will feel more like a partnership, making it more enjoyable for everyone. So go through the recipes on the Foods Four Thought website with your child and see what looks or sounds tasty. You can also plan some fun themed nights for food such as breakfast for dinner, taco salad, outdoor grill, soup night, slow-cooker, stir-fry night, and so on.

Your action item is now to look at the meals from the recipe pages or any others that you might select for a solid week. Make a list of easy snacks you know your child will enjoy when hungry. Designate about two hours on two separate days apart from one another, such as Sunday and Thursday, on which you will do your meal prep. Prepare the first 3–4 meals on the first day, and the remaining meals on the second day. Set a start date for the diet and communicate that information with anyone who will need to know. Clean your kitchen and get rid of any non-conducive food items from your pantry and fridge. Within this time, you will either eat, donate, or toss these foods. Then, it will be time to go shopping. Check off the completed items and answer the questions on the following page. This will help you maintain structure as you prepare to start the diet.

ACTION ITEMS

☐ Browse recipes at the end of this book

☐ Browse other recipes on the FFT website and those listed in the Resources section

What FFT approved snacks does my child like right now? (fruit, nuts, meat, etc.)

_____

_____

_____

What days am I able to meal prep?
Select *two* apart from each other if possible.

(M) (Tu) (W) (Th) (F) (Sa) (Su)

What time will consistently work best for meal prep?

_____

What date will I clean out my pantry? _____

What date will I go grocery shopping? _____

What date will I do our first meal prep? _____

What date will we start the diet? _____

CHAPTER 8

PHASES OF THE DIET

Let's now discuss these first few months as you get your child, and hopefully household, eating only the foods we've talked about and prepared for. Knowing what to expect within the different phases of the diet will help you move forward with confidence.

Phase One: Weeks 1–2
Getting Started

When I first placed my son on the Foods Four Thought Diet, he was like most kids, especially those with a sensory processing disorder. He was not happy about trying new things and giving up the creamy yogurt and graham crackers he loved so much. But I knew this diet was in his very best interest. Thus, we started with what I believed I could get him to try. On day one, this included some cooked chicken, carrots, and celery. Because of his sensory sensitivity, I threw it all in a blender and puréed it. With a bit of salt and Italian seasoning, it wasn't half bad, and he was just barely willing to eat it.

If you're like most parents who crack open this book feeling concerned that your child will be too picky and not agreeable to eat exactly what's on the provided meal plan, it's okay. Trust yourself and feed them what you think they will eat from the four food groups. If that is some homemade applesauce and mashed up carrots in the first week, just go with that and introduce as you go. Again, if the list of foods they will eat is small, try to incorporate more calories by using natural fats blended or cooked into the food. These add good flavor and caloric energy.

An amazing thing happens as your child moves forward on this diet. They will begin eating things you never thought possible. Within one month of being strict on the diet, my son's repertoire of food he was willing to eat tripled. He is not alone. This is in our human nature. When we completely understand that something is no longer available, our neuroplasticity allows us to branch out and find new things to replace that item with. Also, the diet heals the gut which in turn heals the brain. That is part of the role and connection of the vagus nerve we discussed earlier. This then leads to a reduction of sensory processing issues, which then promotes the child's willingness to explore new tastes, textures, smells, and appearances with their food.

You might still think, *No way, not my kid*, but they really will try new foods if you are consistent and positive, and they will be the foods that are approved on this diet. Eating is such a natural instinct, and when we're hungry enough, we eat what's available. We've all experienced this to some degree; you're crazy hungry, but the only thing you can get your hands on is a raw bell pepper stick, and suddenly that's the best bell pepper you've ever tasted in your life. A similar thing happens with most of our kids. Your child may resist for the first little while and only eat a few things they are comfortable with, this is a given. But it will get easier with time. There are a few extreme cases when a problematic eater truly won't eat what they don't want, but again, this is rare. Don't let this fear be an excuse not to give the diet your best effort if your child resists at first.

I recommend picking out a few foods that are FFT approved and keeping them available to eat so your child does not go hungry if they are resistant to the meals. Their diet may seem limited at first if they are unwilling to try anything else. However, as you stick with the process you will see positive things happen as your child slowly but surely begins to experiment with the food provided. If this is just watermelon, applesauce, salted cashews, and some grilled chicken, so be it. You're off to the races. As you move forward, you will diversify your child's diet with a balanced array of the four food groups.

Track Calories

Through this process, especially in the beginning, you must exercise caution and make sure your child is getting enough calories during the day. To achieve this, you can visit health.gov where you can find charts to help you know your child's calorie goals—based on their gender, age, and activity level. I also encourage you to plug their food intake into one of many free calorie trackers such as MyPlate, YAZIO, or Fitbit and gauge how they're doing. Journal this information daily. Try to stay close to the recommended calorie guideline offered by health.gov to remain within a safe range for your child.

100% Dedicated

I'll remind you that it's imperative to stick to the diet with 100% accuracy to see the full results the Foods Four Thought Diet can provide. This is because of the pathogens that feed off of undigested carbohydrates. Eating a food item that is not allowed while on the diet will cause a refeed of those bacteria and fungi, thus prolonging their life and havoc with the intestine.

Experimenting with Foods

If you find that a certain food is not providing the desired effect, such as a specific nut seems to cause abdominal cramping, or eggs are causing hives, keep that food out for at least the next four weeks before trying it in small quantities again. Be alert and journal your child's behaviors and reactions to certain foods. If a particular food seems to cause a severe allergic reaction that is life-threatening such as restricted airways, avoid that food entirely. Though, you are likely aware of any such reactions to a certain food prior to even starting this diet.

Keep trying to add new foods into your child's diet. If they were aversive to pears in week one, give them another try in week three. Their new willingness to give certain foods a go may surprise you. Also, continue to make food fun with themed dinner nights and playing with their food. That's right! Allowing your child to have more tactile experiences may help with any existing food aversions. Plop some oiled and salted zoodles on their plate and encourage them to make fun spiral designs. This can consequently result in taste testing. At the very least, if they will engage in this, it's a sensory win.

Tricks of the Trade

Here are several tips and ideas to help get your picky eater to experiment more with food.

Idea #1: Have them try new foods away from the kitchen. For example, place a new fruit, veggie, or snack in their lap while they are watching a movie or driving in the car. <u>Make sure that it is cut into tiny pieces that they cannot possibly choke on</u>. Their moderate distraction and inclined desire to snack might just open up a whole new menu item.

Idea #2: Pack snacks or meals and eat them somewhere new such as a park or picnic area. Being outdoors is tremendously therapeutic. Additionally, you are away from the kitchen so there are typically no other food options other than what is with you at that moment.

Idea #3: Make sure your child is eating at only specific times. These should be spaced at least two hours apart. They will be more inclined to eat new foods if they are legitimately hungry.

Idea #4: If your child responds to rewards, you could create a star chart. For example, when they try a new food this will equal one star. Once they have tried five new foods, and thus received five stars, they will get a prize, or something along those lines. Make it easy for them to obtain this goal at first, then slowly inch up what is expected of them. Perhaps more bites of those foods, or six new foods instead of five, etc. Always encourage them with positivity and enthusiasm.

Detox Side Effects

It's important to note that occasionally negative side-effects associated with detoxification can pop up within these first two weeks. It does not happen for all, but sometimes this is displayed as headaches, increased aggression, or distractibility. This is normal and can be a sign that things are moving in the right direction. As the pathogens die off, they release their gasses into the system at a rapid rate, whereas before it was a steady rate. There is no imminent danger to this, mainly just an unpleasant child for a few days. But once your child is over this initial hump, it will be far better sailing afterward. This means the bulk of the toxins have left the body, and real recovery can begin. These symptoms will clear up after about two weeks. Occasionally, there is a random flare-up as healing continues, but stay the course, allowing your child to eat only those items that promote healing and journal everything that occurs and is eaten.

I'll reiterate that if you are concerned about how much you think your child will eat or is eating, you are welcome and encouraged to consult your doctor before and during the diet.

So, before you begin week one, you'll start strong, having made your plans clear for the diet with your child, family, friends, and any other caretakers. You will have stocked up at the grocery store and done a major food prep according to the provided 1-week meal plan or based on what you are comfortable presenting your child. These first few weeks will be challenging, but you've got this!

Phase Two: Weeks 3–8
Remember Why You Started

These next several weeks will be all about continuing your journey. You will maintain your routine of shopping, meal prep, plus food and behavior journaling. I differentiate these weeks in the diet from the previous ones, not because the diet itself changes, but because goals and new behaviors typically start to dwindle around this point. Consider the many New Year's resolutions that are forsaken by the time February rolls around. Remembering *why* you started this journey will be imperative at this moment in the program.

At the beginning of week three, I encourage you to take some time and fill out the following goal sheet. We'll use the tried and true acronym SMART to guide us through setting goals and reestablishing what you hope to accomplish through the Foods Four Thought Diet.

S — Specific: Get detailed with your goal. No general wants.
Example: *I want my son to improve his eye contact. Currently, he looks at me when he wants something. I want him to also look at me when we play.*

Example: *I want my daughter to be able to sit through her entire history class without wandering or excessive fidgeting.*

M — Measurable: Trackable progress. Something you can see. This will be easily done if you are regularly keeping your food journal updated.
Example: *I want my child's eczema to clear up by week nine of our strict adherence to the diet.*
Example: *I want my son's diarrhea to clear up by February.*

A — Attainable: Is your goal realistic within the setting? Expecting your child to eliminate their diagnosis through *any* therapy is not reasonable and does everyone a disservice. Rather, look for smaller things that improve their quality of life.
Example: *I want my daughter to use her toys appropriately when playing with her sister.*
Example: *I want my child's teeth grinding to stop.*

R — Relevant: Does your goal align with other parts of your life? This one likely coincides with your overall personal goals. Bettering your child's health naturally improves your ability to obtain other aspirations in your life.

T — Time-bound: Have a date that progress can be measured against. This one is also built into the nature of the diet. As mentioned before, give the diet your all for at least two months. If you have seen no progress within that time you may need to seek out other forms of therapy or more restrictive diets. If you have seen some progress and feel more is to come, stay strict to the four primary food groups discussed earlier.

Setting goals for your child should not be taken lightly. We can never have full control over what progress they experience. We can only do our part to educate ourselves and put the work in from our end. If the goals you set here are not met within your time frame, take heart. It is nothing to blame yourself or your child for. It simply means it is not the time for such progress. Contemplating reasonable goals you have for your child as they work through the diet will help motivate you to maintain the rules of eating within the approved foods list.

Now, take a quiet moment and fill in the question on the next page. Keep in mind the SMART guidelines. Maintain positivity as you answer the question. This is not a time for mourning what is not yet had. Rather, you are considering the possibility of what milestones might present themselves as the result of a refreshed body and mind.

ASPIRED GOALS

Name three things you hope your child will achieve as a result of improved health.

1) _____
   _____
   _____

2) _____
   _____
   _____

3) _____
   _____
   _____

Regardless of whether these goals are met within the next two to twelve months of strictly adhering to the FFT Diet, you should be proud. Proud of the work you and your child have put in to obtain better health. I do not doubt that by the end of week eight you will have witnessed several improvements as a result of eating in this healthful way. In week nine I will encourage you to make a similar list, but with improvements that were actually made. We'll visit this in the next section.

Lastly, as I've mentioned before, your child is already incredible. Setting goals is not intended to take away from where they're at this moment. We appreciate where they are and who they are, with a mind toward a positive possibility. We still find joy and gratitude in the present for all things.

Phase Three: Weeks 9+
Reintroduction

Making the Decision

Let's now discuss the reintroduction you may want to consider by the time you reach week nine. As I've mentioned before, two months is the absolute minimum amount of time your child will need to determine if the diet is effective for them. After this point, it is up to you to decide how to proceed. You can remain strictly committed to the diet and watch as further healing and behavior benefits unfold, or you can begin slowly introducing healthy new foods one at a time and watch for symptoms.

As was mentioned earlier, the diet was so incredible for our son that we strictly adhered to the FFT Diet rules for four years before reintroducing foods such as quinoa, beans, and healthier forms of dairy. So for four Thanksgiving celebrations, I was toting our own safe little Tupperware meal to our families' houses. For four years, my kids traded in their Halloween candy at the end of trick-or-treating for the toys my husband and I had purchased them. For four years, my son had his favorite chicken strips on his birthday and a delicious diet-approved cake from the comfort of our home. And for four years, my son's body was allowed the peace it required to rest, reset, and rebuild. By that time, he had gained his best health, and we never again saw a food allergy or even an aversive behavior afterward—not once!

So again, this part is up to you. Do you feel the diet is working but needs more time? For this, you would stay the course and stick to the foods from the four pillars; vegetables, fruit, healthy fats, and animal proteins. You can then carefully experiment when you feel the time is right. Or, are you ready to start introducing safe food choices to see how your child fares? This would mean you start including mild, starchy vegetables or grains. If you're unsure what to do, I heartily suggest taking some time to sit quietly and listen to your intuitive self. This is the power you hold and it should not be undermined. You know what your child needs over and above anyone else. This decision is yours.

Reintroduction

Once you decide to begin reintroducing foods—whether that's after eight weeks or eight months—you will do this slowly and deliberately, testing each food one at a time. With each new food that is added, watch for any aversions either physical or behavioral. If you find that a food causes a negative reaction, you will journal it and not introduce that food again for at least another month.

You will also want to wait at least four days between introducing new foods. So if you introduce a yam on Monday, wait until Friday before you try quinoa, and so on. Four days is enough time to see if there is a negative reaction to a food. You do not want an overlap because you might think one food is the culprit for a stomach ache or a rash, when in fact it was a different food that was introduced.

Also, when introducing a new food, start in small quantities, such as a teaspoon or tablespoon portion. If your child tolerates it, you can move to a slightly larger size on the following day and so on. It may take up to four days for a symptom to appear, so keep portions small during these first few days. If there have been no negative physical or behavioral setbacks after four days, the food is likely tolerated and can be included in their daily diet.

The following chart lists the stages to introduce certain foods. The foods in each category are in no particular order, and all possibilities are not listed. This is just to lend you a good idea for what types of foods you can look to reintroduce first.

Reintroduction Stage 1	Beans, Brown rice, Chia seeds, Corn, Flax seeds, Lentils, Oats, Peas, Potatoes, Plantains, Quinoa, Yams
Reintroduction Stage 2	Goat milk, Maple syrup, Mushrooms, Stevia, Tomatoes
Reintroduction Stage 3 These should really be omitted on a daily basis. However, it may be good to know your child's response to these foods. Introduce carefully, note reactions. If tolerated, eat sparingly. Always find the most natural source of these products (ie. organic, nonGMO, etc.).	Cane Sugar Casein products — Cheese, Milk, Yogurt Gluten products — Barley, Rye, Buckwheat, Wheat Soy products — Tempeh, Tofu, Soybean oil (nonGMO)

Again, by the ninth week, you have allowed enough time to see if the diet is, in fact, valuable for your child. When you decide to reintroduce food—be it eight weeks or eight months after your start date—you will gain powerful knowledge as to what foods your child can truly tolerate. Though I'll reiterate that I absolutely recommend staying as close to these four food groups in their natural state as often as possible now and forever after. These foods will allow for the best possible bodily function throughout the lifetime, which is something we all need more of.

Now, take a quiet moment at the start of week nine and fill in the questions on the next page. As you answer these you will be guided with the knowledge on how to proceed. This may include staying the course within the four main food groups, or perhaps a slow reintroduction. Again, maintain positivity as you answer the questions and own confidence that you hold the answer to what your child needs at this time.

REFLECTIVE QUESTIONS

Name at least three health improvements your child has made over the last eight weeks, either physical, mental or emotional.

1) _____
   _____

2) _____
   _____

3) _____
   _____

What does your gut tell you about the reintroduction of new foods? Do you want to branch out at this time? Why or why not?

_____
_____
_____
_____
_____
_____

Foods Four Thought Diet

CHAPTER 9

ADDITIONAL TOOLS

Planning for Parties and School

Parties and classroom events can be daunting for *anyone* adhering to a restrictive diet, whether it's for health or simple weight loss. However, making the diet work outside of the safety of your home is possible with a bit of planning and communication. No reclusion is required.

Here are a few common places you may encounter for which you must armor up with Tupperware or a lunchbox full of delicious, healthy food.

- Daycare
- Grandma's house
- Holiday/Birthday party
- School
- Restaurant meetup
- A long day out

If your child goes to school or daycare, prepping meals for lunch won't be too difficult, especially if you're already sending them to school with a home lunch. You'll have to make sure all the packed food is FFT approved, and that there is plenty of it. Also, I don't recommend getting too creative with school lunches. Stick to their preferred foods that you are confident they will eat and that are approved.

You'll want to make sure that the teacher is aware of your dietary intentions and new strict rules around food. You can download a pre-written letter for your child's teacher at www.foodsfourthought.com/teacher-letter. You can edit and send this to the educator before your family begins the diet. Also, ask that the teacher share this information with other pertinent staff, such as those who might attend lunch with the class. This way they can help ensure your child is not eating or exchanging non-approved food items with classmates.

Before school or events, remind your child why you all are embarking on this diet using the charting and communication printouts previously mentioned. If you are using the calendar, remind them of their need to eat only the food you send them to school with if they want the reward at the end of the predetermined period. If they require less support or are older and used the checklist, remind them that the diet is meant to help them feel and function better, so they will need to eat only the healthy food you provide. These tools will help them make good decisions while they are out of your vision.

School parties are where it gets tricky. However, the same protocol should be followed. As you will see in the teacher letter, they should contact you if there is a party, allowing you time to plan accordingly. You can then send the child to school with a second lunch to eat in the event of a classroom function. It may seem harsh to have your child pass on a pizza party, but just remember, they are not likely the only kid in the classroom who must avoid certain foods. The prevalence of food allergies is significantly higher than ever before. I have found there is always at least one or two other children in a classroom of thirty kids with food sensitivities. These children also have to make alternative dietary preparations. Remind your child that this level of strict food adherence is temporary and their current sacrifices will help them gain better health or that prize awaiting them.

Sometimes a child will randomly bring treats to class. To combat this, you will provide the teacher with a labeled bag and your child's name on it. This will contain approved snacks for your child so they will have something to eat that is healthy and preferred. You can ask the teacher to keep these snacks in a designated cupboard. This is also addressed in the teacher letter. You can find several pre-packaged snacks that are FFT approved at www.foodsfourthought.com/products.

The same goes for holiday celebrations and birthday parties. If there is a birthday party, consider making your child's favorite approved food and treat. I definitely suggest the chocolate cake listed towards the latter part of the recipe pages. It's so rich and tasty; they won't feel like they are missing out. If you are vegan, or want a tasty alternative, you can make the chocolate almond fruit dip in the dessert section. This is delicious with fresh sliced apples. For traditional dinner spreads, you can substitute mashed potatoes for mashed cauliflower. If there are rolls, make some No-Cornbread from the snack section of the recipe pages. If there is pudding at the party, make the Berries and Cream, or find a chocolate pudding recipe from the Foods Four Thought website. There really are so many alternatives to traditional dishes that are nutritious and delicious.

Now, about those lovely family gatherings. These can be one of the most challenging aspects for some who are embarking on a lifestyle change. This will not consistently be true for all. But for others, family members that do not shy away from questions and criticism can be a frustrating reality. If you suspect running into this, you'll want to consider coming prepared with your convictions that your child needs this dietary intervention right now. You could even share a bit about what you've learned regarding the link between disorders and diet, and leave it at that. Be respectful of the fact that most people are trying to be helpful, though once in a while we are graced with a diehard pessimist who genuinely looks to discredit anyone's ideas. These individuals are fortunately the lesser common. Just remember to be courteous, kind, and certain that you are taking the right action. No one can get you down if this remains your attitude and outlook.

Organization

Having peace of mind within your home is an important element and will help you maintain dietary organization and positivity through the process. For many on the outside looking in, staying organized seems like it should be straightforward. But for those of us with families, jobs, and extracurricular events, remaining organized can be overwhelming. And while organization is important, it does not have to be on complete lockdown before you start the diet. Instead, start small and consider dedicating fifteen minutes each day to declutter or deep clean one small area of your home. Try to make it happen at the same time each day, such as after cleaning up from dinner. This will better ensure that it gets done. Bins, bags, and folders go a long way to help organize drawers and cupboards. Even zip-lock bags can be great because items remain contained and you can toss objects in those that apply to each other.

Another tidy-home-tip learned over the years is the acronym "OHIO." This stands for Only Handle It Once—meaning if you touch it, you put it away, don't set it down somewhere it does not finally belong. This term is easy to remember and helps prevent the accumulation of clutter all over floors and tables throughout the day. When house members have something in-hand, they can remember to get it to its proper place, not just to the nearest surface.

Next, make a weekly to-do list. You could complete this after you have done your meal planning for the week. Arrange these items in order of importance, this will help ensure that the most urgent tasks get done first. You may also want to give your items a designated day for completion such as Monday: Change batteries in the smoke detector, Tuesday: Mow the lawn—and so on. This allows tasks to feel more obtainable and will better ensure you don't overestimate how much you can get done in one day. Check this to-do list daily. The first thing in the morning may be an optimal time for this.

It is also a good idea to keep a notepad or digital task list handy which will allow you to jot down ideas or chores that require addressing later. Check these items off as you complete them. This will promote a sense of accomplishment, which is important as you move through your week. Another tip that can help encourage emotional health is to write down the things you accomplished, even if they were not on your original checklist. Often our days get ahead of us and by the end, we feel as though we couldn't get anything done we aspired to do. These feelings promote a negative perception of self, when in reality we do many things every day. Thus, towards the end of the day take a few moments to write down all that you accomplished—such as making your way through the Everest of laundry, picking up your dog's meds, and so on. This will help appease those gnawing feelings of guilt and inadequacy.

It is also important to keep your calendar up to date and again, check it daily. This will avoid feelings of stress as you will be well-prepared for upcoming events and can plan accordingly. Also, do not allow yourself to feel bogged down with events that do not require your attendance such as your neighbor's niece's wedding. If you don't want to go, then don't. If it's not a mandatory event, do not push or stress yourself to make it to functions that can overcrowd your schedule. Doing so can detract from your overall goals.

Last, do not buy unneeded items. This will not only save your home from clutter but will also save your bank account. Minor items can add up in a big way. Instead, go through your home and gather up items you no longer have use for. Create a timeline for this, depending on the item. If you haven't used it in 1–2 years, it's likely safe to toss, donate, or sell.

Overcoming Obstacles and Negativity

Throughout our life, we will find many moments when remaining positive within our circumstances is paramount. Raising young children with unique challenges is one of such situations. When we embark on something new and important, no matter what it is, feeling a lack of support from certain people in our life is frequently just part of the equation. Often this is not because that person or the surrounding people want you to fail, it may be they are afraid that your efforts will not yield your expectations. But in the words of Albert Einstein, "You never fail until you stop trying." Supporting your child from the inside out is a process. It takes time and there will be trials, that's a guarantee, but the intent is that the outcome will be worth it for your child and the family. Fortunately, the research also points towards this end.

Aside from your own doubts and questions of adequacy, you will likely have to deal with nay-sayers. These may be people in your immediate or distant family, friends, neighbors, or coworkers. You will need to see past that curtain of negativity and keep moving forward in your own journey. Your decisions are based on what you know to be in the best interest of your family. Oftentimes friction regarding changes in the household comes from a significant other. This is difficult and stressful, to say the least. The best thing to do in this situation is to reach out to a supportive group of people or a singular person who can identify with your course of action and support your endeavor. You can also join the Foods Four Thought Support Community Facebook Group. Here, we bolster each other and it is a safe space to post concerns, questions, and receive simple but much-needed emotional aid.

Self-Care

You-Time – Considering your critical role as a caretaker to a child with unique needs, it's crucial that your self-care does not fall by the wayside. It is imperative that you receive the time you need to find moments of pure peace and relaxation. This can look different from person to person. You may find rejuvenation through a morning hike, an hour at the spa, a completed project, a date night, or simply time alone. Whatever respite looks like for you, find a way to make time for it. This can feel like a tall order, especially if you still have small children at home. But finding yourself amongst the daily to-do's, and reconnecting with yourself and your desires is so tremendously important to your physical and emotional health.

If you are the extreme selfless caretaker type, it will be difficult for you to imagine taking time for yourself. However, remember that your loved ones need you to be running at your optimal. The only way to do this is to find time to rejuvenate at least once per week on a deep level. I suggest finding a relaxing activity and making arrangements that allow you at least one full hour to yourself or with people whose company you truly value.

Meditation – Outside of the one hour "You-Time," it will also be important to connect with yourself through daily meditation. This can be anywhere from 5 to 30 minutes. You can do this with the use of relaxing music, a guided meditation, or pure silence. It does not have to be fancy. Just a quiet moment and space where you allow yourself the love, peace, and acceptance you deserve. Meditation is such a powerful tool that allows us to know ourselves, our intentions, and everything around us so much more clearly.

Listed here are several clinically researched benefits of meditation to help motivate you to include it in your daily life if you haven't done so already.

- Improved problem-solving
- Improved stress resilience
- Improved self-compassion
- Improved emotional intelligence

Exercise – Exercise is also a powerful self-care tool. Physical activity is often muddied as something that is used to help us look externally better. And while this may be an additional perk, it is far from the main accomplishment of exercise. Physical activity improves our health on a cellular level and improves our coordination, joint pain, critical organs, and sleep—just to name a few physical benefits. It is also extremely powerful at helping us manage our mental and emotional health through our bodies' release of endorphins. This chemical delivery helps us manage stress, minimize depression, and improve our self-confidence.

Exercise does not have to look like hitting the gym for sixty minutes per day. It can come in whatever form you feel most uplifted by. This can include gardening, hiking, walking, running, tennis, group classes, weight lifting, or yoga. The best physical activity is anything that gets your heart pumping and makes you feel accomplished and elevated. Try to fit any preferred exercises into your schedule for 20–30 minutes, 3–7 days per week.

I encourage you now to take some time and set up a self-care schedule for the upcoming week. Make sure to include a minimum of 30 minutes of self-care every single day. Below is an example of what yours might look like. Be sure to include at the very least three days of exercise, three days of meditation, and one day of anything you want to spend an hour doing that feeds a special level of yourself either socially, emotionally, or creatively. Write your schedule down and chip away at making your self-care a priority.

Example Self-Care Schedule

Monday — Exercise: Gym, 6 am
Tuesday — Meditate, 6 am
Wednesday — Exercise: Trail walk with a friend, 6 am
Thursday — Meditate, 6 am
Friday — Exercise: Garden, 6 am
Saturday — Date Night, 5 pm
Sunday — Meditate, 6 am

MY SELF-CARE SCHEDULE

Monday
_____

Tuesday
_____

Wednesday
_____

Thursday
_____

Friday
_____

Saturday
_____

Sunday
_____

CHAPTER 10

A FINAL WORD

Within only a few months, you will have committed to and accomplished something incredible. Your dedication and sacrifice will change the way you and your family see food. You will know that food, if wielded well, is a powerful tool for self-defense, health, and personal care.

The remainder of this book will be used to provide you with additional knowledge and to make the diet free of guesswork. You may be required to problem-solve based on the individual needs of your child and household, but the tools ahead will help to make that as seamless as possible.

Remember to join the Foods Four Thought Support Community Facebook Group. Here you will have access to myself to help you navigate questions or concerns, as well as other caretakers who are venturing through the diet as well.

It is my sincere desire that you have gained light and knowledge through these pages. That your thirst to obtain health for yourself and your family will continue well beyond this singular diet. My love and well-wishes are with you and your family.

Warmest regards always,
Crystal

CHAPTER 11

IN THE KITCHEN AND RECIPES

Glycemic Index of Fruit

Here is a brief look at a few low and medium glycemic index (GI) fruits. Higher GI fruits in the Medium column are still excellent and can certainly be consumed but keep them in moderation with the rest of the food on the diet.

LOW		**MEDIUM**	
Apples	Citrus fruits	Banana	Papaya
Apricot	Peaches	Grapes	Pineapples
Berries	Pears	Dates	Mango
Cherries	Plum	Kiwi	Watermelon

Substitution Chart

No	Yes
Butter	Coconut oil or Ghee
Flour	Almond or Coconut flour*
Milk	Almond or Coconut milk**
Peanut butter	Almond, Cashew, or Sesame butter
Soy sauce	Coconut aminos
Sugar	Coconut or Date sugar
Wheat noodles	Zoodles or Spaghetti squash
Vegetable oil	Olive, Coconut, or Avocado oil

*You cannot make a straight swap of wheat flour for almond or coconut flour. Coconut flour is extremely dry, while almond flour is more wet. Making this swap will take some getting used to if the recipe does not already call for it. However, the general rules of thumb are:

- Use 50% more almond flour than a wheat flour recipe calls for, and 50% less liquid. (i.e. a recipe calls for 1 cup of wheat flour and 1/2 cup of milk. You use 1.5 cups of almond flour and 1/4 cup of coconut milk)
- Use 1/3 cup of coconut flour to every 1 cup of wheat flour, plus 1 egg. If it is still too thick, consider adding one more egg or coconut and almond milk until the desired consistency is achieved.
- If a gluten-free batter seems too runny, it will likely not bake well. This is unlike a wheat cake recipe which is commonly runny. If you choose to modify your favorite traditional recipes, you will inevitably go through some trial and error—thus experiment in small quantities.

** Most store-bought milk will contain ingredients that are not approved within the first phase of the diet. Thus, shop carefully or make your own. You can buy a plant-based milk maker for around $200. This is an investment but many find it's well worth it. I've listed it on the Products page of the Foods Four Thought website.

Kitchen Must-Haves

Appliances
- ☐ Food processor
- ☐ Powerful blender
- ☐ Instant pot
- ☐ Slow cooker (not necessary if your Instant pot has this feature)
- ☐ Electric mixer
- ☐ Griddle
- ☐ Waffle iron (not necessary, but nice for a change)
- ☐ Plant-based milk maker (not necessary, but nice to have)

Utensils
- ☐ Vegetable peeler
- ☐ Tongs
- ☐ Kitchen scissors
- ☐ Rubber spatula
- ☐ Soup ladle
- ☐ Cookie Scoop

Basics
- ☐ Pots and pans, various sizes
- ☐ Measuring cups and spoons
- ☐ Baking sheet

- ☐ Muffin tin
- ☐ Cutting boards (1 for meat and 1 for vegetables)
- ☐ Strainer
- ☐ Glass storage containers, various sizes
- ☐ Mixing bowls, various sizes
- ☐ Parchment paper
- ☐ Large salad bowl

1–Week Shopping List

Listed on the following pages are all of the ingredients you'll need for the recipes within the 1-week meal plan. These items will get you through the week of recipes and additional snacks. The highlighted rows will typically not need to be purchased weekly, rather bi-weekly or less, depending on the product. As a result, the first week will be the most expensive if you do not already have the listed foods on hand. However, later weeks should be significantly less costly. For example:

- Shopping cost Week 1— $483
- Shopping cost Week 2— $193

I've included pricing in this list to help you gauge expenses if that's something you regularly track. Prices are of course subject to change depending on your global location, time of year, or individual retailer.

Refrigerator/Freezer		
Item	**Quantity**	**Cost**
Eggs	40	$12
Ghee	14 oz	$11
Almond milk	32 fl oz	$3
Orange juice	52 fl oz	$4
Apple juice	52 fl oz	$4
Frozen pineapple	10 oz	$3
Frozen mixed berries	5 lb	$14
Frozen strawberries	10 oz	$3

Spices		
Item	**Quantity**	**Cost**
Cinnamon	10 oz	$4
Nutmeg	1 oz	$6
Salt	10 oz	$4
Pepper	2 oz	$4
Italian seasoning	1 oz	$4
Paprika	1.6 oz	$6
Cumin	1.5 oz	$4

Foods Four Thought Diet

Ground ginger	1.5 oz		$4
Turmeric	2 oz		$4
Dried thyme	1 oz		$7
Curry powder	1.5 oz		$3
Chili powder	2 oz		$3
Dried oregano	0.5 oz		$3
Dried parsley	0.2 oz		$3
Dried basil	0.5 oz		$5
Mustard seed	1.5 oz		$2
Poppy seeds	2 oz		$6
Sesame seeds	1.3 oz		$5

Produce		
Item	**Quantity**	**Cost**
Strawberries	2 lbs	$8
Blueberries	18 oz	$7
Peaches	5 lbs	$12
Apples	5.5 lbs	$16
Bananas	1 bunch	$3
Orange	1 item	$2

Mandaries	3 items	$2
Lime	3 items	$2
Avocado	2 items	$4
Carrots	2 lbs	$7
Celery	1 bunch	$3
Garlic	1 bulb	$1
Red bell peppers	7 items	$14
Yellow bell peppers	1 item	$2
Orange bell peppers	1 item	$2
Green bell peppers	1 item	$1
Green onions	2 bunches	$2
Sweet onions	10 lbs	$11
Leek	1 bunch	$4
Red leaf lettuce	4 heads	$8
Spinach	32 oz	$10
Asparagus	2 lbs	$7
Cilantro	2 bunches	$2

Interior Isles		
Item	**Quantity**	**Cost**
Olive oil	4 L	$21
Honey	3 lb	$12
Balsamic vinegar	17 fl oz	$7
Apple cider vinegar	16 oz	$4
Dijon mustard	12 oz	$2
Yellow mustard	9 oz	$4
Coconut oil	84 oz	$13
Coconut flour	1 lb	$11
Coconut milk	5 cans	$15
Coconut aminos	8 fl oz	$7
Coconut nectar (if vegan)	12 fl oz	$7
Coconut sugar	3 lbs	$14
Baking soda	16 oz	$1
Shredded coconut	8 oz	$3
Almond butter	27 oz	$10
Tahini	16 oz	$6
Pumpkin	1—15 oz can	$3

Cacao powder	1 lb	$11
Olives	6.5 fl oz	$2
Raisins	12 oz	$4
Dates	10 oz.	$5
Pecans	2 lbs	$15
Walnuts	3 lbs	$12
Cashews	16 oz	$8
Almonds	2.5 lbs	$15
Almonds, slivered	2 lbs	$10

1- WEEK MEAL PLAN

	BREAKFAST	LUNCH	SNACK	DINNER	
MONDAY	Blueberry Muffins & Applesauce pg. 123 & 139	Energy Bites & Cooked Carrots pg. 137	Nuts, Leftovers, Cooked or Raw Fruits or Vegetables	Tahini Salad & Spiced Cream Soup pg. 151 & 153	
TUESDAY	Smoothie & Pecan Cookies pg. 125 & 133	Blueberry Muffins & Applesauce pg. 123 & 139	Nuts, Leftovers, Cooked or Raw Fruits or Vegetables	Vinaigrette Salad & Asparagus Soup pg. 155 & 157	
WEDNESDAY	Banana Cake & Applesauce pg. 129 & 139	Pecan Cookies & Peaches pg. 133	Nuts, Leftovers, Cooked or Raw Fruits or Vegetables	Lime Cilantro Salad Vegetable Chili pg. 159 & 161	
THURSDAY	Smoothie Bowl & Granola pg. 133 & 141	Banana Cake & Ants on Log pg. 137	Nuts, Leftovers, Cooked or Raw Fruits or Vegetables	Poppyseed Salad Pumpkin Soup pg. 163 & 165	
FRIDAY	Strawberry Muffins & Applesauce pg. 127 & 139	Energy Bites & Cooked Carrots pg. 137	Nuts, Leftovers, Cooked or Raw Fruits or Vegetables	Curried Salad & Creamy Curry Soup pg 167 & 169	
SATURDAY	Smoothie & Granola pg. 133 & 141	Strawberry Muffins & Pears pg. 135	Nuts, Leftovers, Cooked or Raw Fruits or Vegetables	Honey Mustard Salad & Creamy Veggie Soup pg. 171 & 173	
SUNDAY	Waffles with Berry Honey Sauce pg. 131	Energy Bites & Cooked Carrots pg. 137	Nuts, Leftovers, Cooked or Raw Fruits or Vegetables	Strawberry Spinach Salad & Red Pepper Soup pg. 175 & 177	

RECIPES

BREAKFAST, 121

LUNCH & SNACKS, 135

DINNER, 148

SWEET TREATS, 179

Foods Four Thought Diet

BREAKFAST

Blueberry Muffins & Pecan Crumble, 123

Coconut Pecan Cookies, 125

Strawberry Banana Muffins, 127

Banana Cake with Crumb Topping, 129

Easy Waffle & Strawberry Syrup, 131

Smoothies, 133

Blueberry Muffins & Pecan Crumble

NUTRITION INFORMATION

Serving Size: 1 Serving

Nutrient	Quantity	Nutrient	Quantity
Calories	428 kcal	Vitamin B-6	0.193 mg
Carbohydrates	31.76 g	Vitamin B-12 (Cobalamin)	3.02 µg
Fiber	2.1 g	Vitamin A	401 IU
Sugars	29.23 g	Vitamin E	1.1 mg
Starch	0.09 g	Vitamin D	39 IU
Total Fat	31.41 g	Vitamin K	3.9 µg
Omega 3	0.177 g	Calcium	54 mg
Omega 6	3.015 g	Magnesium	31 mg
Monounsaturated Fat	8.667 g	Phosphorus	162 mg
Protein	8.68 g	Iron	2.74 mg
Vitamin C	1.5 mg	Potassium	270 mg
Folate	49 µg	Sodium	178 mg
Vitamin B-1 (Thiamin)	0.179 mg	Zinc	1.34 mg
Vitamin B-2 (Riboflavin)	0.29 mg	Copper	0.199 mg
Vitamin B-3 (Niacin)	0.33 mg	Selenium	21.3 µg
Vitamin B-5 (Pantothenic acid)	1.198 mg	Manganese	0.628 mg

BLUEBERRY MUFFINS & PECAN CRUMBLE

SERVES	PREP TIME	COOK TIME	READY IN
5	15 min	15 min	30 min

ALLERGENS: coconut, eggs, pecans

NOTES: These muffins are so satisfying and just sweet enough that you feel content without the guilt. They are a perfect morning start or an afternoon pick me up.

INGREDIENTS

- 4 eggs
- 1/4 cup honey
- 1/4 cup coconut oil, melted *
- 1/2 cup coconut flour
- 1/2 tsp baking soda
- 1/2 tsp apple cider vinegar
- Dash of salt
- 1 cup fresh blueberries

Crumble

- 1/2 cup pecans, chopped
- 2 Tbsp coconut flour
- 2 Tbsp coconut sugar
- 2 Tbsp coconut oil, melted
- Dash of salt

*Coconut oil should be barely melted, not hot. Adding hot oil to eggs will scramble them.

DIRECTIONS

1. Preheat oven to 350 °F. Line a standard muffin pan with coconut oil or paper liners.
2. In a medium glass bowl, using an electric mixer, mix eggs until blended. Add honey and mix until combined. Slowly add in the melted coconut oil*. Mix in coconut flour and salt until smooth. Add in the baking soda and vinegar. Mix until just blended.
3. Fold the fresh blueberries into the batter.
4. Divide the batter between the 10 muffin molds. Pat down as needed.
5. In a separate small glass bowl, combine all crumble ingredients. Sprinkle evenly over the muffins.
6. Bake in the preheated oven for 15 minutes or until the edges are brown and muffins are cooked through.

Coconut Pecan Cookies

NUTRITION INFORMATION

Serving Size: 1 Serving

Nutrient	Quantity	Nutrient	Quantity
Calories	216 kcal	Vitamin B-6	0.109 mg
Carbohydrates	19.8 g	Vitamin B-12 (Cobalamin)	1.89 µg
Fiber	0.8 g	Vitamin A	239 IU
Sugars	18.66 g	Vitamin E	0.53 mg
Starch	0.02 g	Vitamin D	24 IU
Total Fat	13.93 g	Vitamin K	0.4 µg
Omega 3	0.062 g	Calcium	36 mg
Omega 6	1.159 g	Magnesium	18 mg
Monounsaturated Fat	3.947 g	Phosphorus	93 mg
Protein	5.06 g	Iron	1.69 mg
Vitamin C	0.9 mg	Potassium	178 mg
Folate	30 µg	Sodium	156 mg
Vitamin B-1 (Thiamin)	0.084 mg	Zinc	0.72 mg
Vitamin B-2 (Riboflavin)	0.171 mg	Copper	0.08 mg
Vitamin B-3 (Niacin)	0.16 mg	Selenium	13.3 µg
Vitamin B-5 (Pantothenic acid)	0.707 mg	Manganese	0.269 mg

COCONUT PECAN COOKIES

SERVES	PREP TIME	COOK TIME	READY IN
8	15 min	12 min	27 min

ALLERGENS: coconut, eggs, pecans

NOTES: These cookies were one of my first FFT creation and continue to be a favorite. Experiment with different add-ins such as seeds, goji berries, etc. and they always turn out awesome.

INGREDIENTS

- 4 eggs
- 1/4 cup coconut oil, softened
- 1/2 cup honey
- 3/4 cup coconut flour
- 1 tsp baking soda
- 1 tsp cinnamon
- 1/4 tsp sea salt
- 1/4 cup shredded coconut, unsweetened
- 1/4 cup pecans, chopped
- 1/2 cup raisins

Makes 24 cookies

DIRECTIONS

1. Preheat your oven to 350 °F. Line a baking sheet with parchment paper.
2. Combine the eggs, oil, and honey with an electric mixer. Mix in the flour, baking soda, cinnamon, and sea salt. Once combined, stir in the shredded coconut, pecans, and raisins.
3. Roll the dough into 1-inch balls and flatten between your hands slightly before placing them on your prepared cookie sheet.
4. Bake for approximately 12 minutes or until the edges and top are barely golden. Drizzle lightly with honey if desired.

Strawberry Banana Muffins

NUTRITION INFORMATION

Serving Size: 1 Serving

Nutrient	Quantity	Nutrient	Quantity
Calories	297 kcal	Vitamin B-6	0.232 mg
Carbohydrates	17.36 g	Vitamin B-12 (Cobalamin)	1.89 µg
Fiber	2.1 g	Vitamin A	252 IU
Sugars	12.95 g	Vitamin E	0.77 mg
Starch	0.87 g	Vitamin D	24 IU
Total Fat	23.72 g	Vitamin K	2.2 µg
Omega 3	1.315 g	Calcium	47 mg
Omega 6	6.014 g	Magnesium	40 mg
Monounsaturated Fat	4.394 g	Phosphorus	137 mg
Protein	7.03 g	Iron	2 mg
Vitamin C	15.8 mg	Potassium	281 mg
Folate	49 µg	Sodium	170 mg
Vitamin B-1 (Thiamin)	0.116 mg	Zinc	1.01 mg
Vitamin B-2 (Riboflavin)	0.193 mg	Copper	0.269 mg
Vitamin B-3 (Niacin)	0.44 mg	Selenium	13.9 µg
Vitamin B-5 (Pantothenic acid)	0.827 mg	Manganese	0.624 mg

STRAWBERRY BANANA MUFFINS

SERVES	PREP TIME	COOK TIME	READY IN
6	15 min	25 min	40 min

ALLERGENS: coconut, eggs, walnuts

NOTES: These muffins are perfect for breakfast and make a great leftover snack. They are soft and perfectly sweetened with the timeless flavor combo of strawberries and bananas.

INGREDIENTS

- 1 banana, very ripe and mashed
- 3 eggs
- 3 Tbsp honey
- 1/4 cup coconut oil, melted*
- 1/2 cup coconut flour
- 1/4 tsp cinnamon
- 1/4 tsp nutmeg
- 1/4 tsp salt
- 1 tsp baking soda
- 1 tsp vinegar
- 1 cup strawberries, chopped
- 1 cup walnuts, chopped

*Coconut oil should be barely melted, not hot. Combining hot oil with the eggs will scramble the eggs.

DIRECTIONS

1. Preheat the oven to 350 °F. Line your muffin tin with 12 paper liners.
2. With an electric mixer combine the banana, eggs, honey, and oil. Add the coconut flour, cinnamon, nutmeg, and salt. Once well mixed add the baking soda and vinegar, combine until just incorporated. Fold in the strawberries and walnuts. Evenly divide the batter between the 12 baking liners.
3. Bake the muffins for 25 minutes or until golden and cooked through.

Banana Cake with Crumb Topping

NUTRITION INFORMATION

Serving Size: 1 Serving

Nutrient	Quantity	Nutrient	Quantity
Calories	187 kcal	Vitamin B-6	0.185 mg
Carbohydrates	17.23 g	Vitamin B-12 (Cobalamin)	1.42 µg
Fiber	1.5 g	Vitamin A	199 IU
Sugars	12.89 g	Vitamin E	0.41 mg
Starch	1.61 g	Vitamin D	18 IU
Total Fat	12.28 g	Vitamin K	0.6 µg
Omega 3	0.032 g	Calcium	34 mg
Omega 6	0.465 g	Magnesium	19 mg
Monounsaturated Fat	2.22 g	Phosphorus	70 mg
Protein	3.91 g	Iron	1.27 mg
Vitamin C	3.2 mg	Potassium	229 mg
Folate	28 µg	Sodium	135 mg
Vitamin B-1 (Thiamin)	0.057 mg	Zinc	0.47 mg
Vitamin B-2 (Riboflavin)	0.144 mg	Copper	0.055 mg
Vitamin B-3 (Niacin)	0.289 mg	Selenium	10.2 µg
Vitamin B-5 (Pantothenic acid)	0.606 mg	Manganese	0.3 mg

BANANA CAKE WITH CRUMB TOPPING

SERVES	PREP TIME	COOK TIME	READY IN
8	15 min	45 min	1 hr

ALLERGENS: coconut, eggs

NOTES: This cake will not have you missing the age-old banana cake or bread you grew up on. It is so delicate, not too sweet, and the crumb topping adds plenty of extra excitement.

INGREDIENTS

- 2 ripe bananas
- 3 eggs
- 3 Tbsp honey
- 1/4 cup coconut oil, melted*
- 1/2 cup coconut flour
- 2 tsp cinnamon
- 1/4 tsp sea salt
- 1 tsp baking soda
- 1 tsp vinegar

Crumble:

- 1 Tbsp coconut oil, melted
- 1/4 cup coconut flour
- 2 Tbsp coconut sugar
- 1 tsp cinnamon

*Coconut oil should be barely melted, not hot. Combining hot oil with the eggs will scramble the eggs.

DIRECTIONS

1. Preheat the oven to 350 °F. Liberally grease an 8 x 8 glass baking dish, or double the recipe and use a 9 x 13 dish.
2. Place the bananas, eggs, honey, and coconut oil into a powerful blender. Combine until smooth. Add in the flour and remaining ingredients. Blend just until combined. Pour into the prepared baking dish.
3. In a small glass bowl combine the crumb topping ingredients and sprinkle evenly over the cake. Bake in the preheated oven for 35 minutes. Turn off the oven and allow the cake to sit in the oven for 10 more minutes. (If the recipe was doubled be sure to increase the cooking time.)
4. Garnish with fresh bananas if desired.

Easy Waffles & Strawberry Syrup

NUTRITION INFORMATION

Serving Size: 1 Serving

Nutrient	Quantity	Nutrient	Quantity
Calories	428 kcal	Vitamin B-6	0.38 mg
Carbohydrates	31.51 g	Vitamin B-12 (Cobalamin)	7.56 µg
Fiber	1.8 g	Vitamin A	969 IU
Sugars	27.52 g	Vitamin E	2.05 mg
Starch	0 g	Vitamin D	97 IU
Total Fat	26.19 g	Vitamin K	2 µg
Omega 3	0.138 g	Calcium	112 mg
Omega 6	1.726 g	Magnesium	36 mg
Monounsaturated Fat	9.541 g	Phosphorus	321 mg
Protein	18.43 g	Iron	6.03 mg
Vitamin C	22.5 mg	Potassium	463 mg
Folate	122 µg	Sodium	230 mg
Vitamin B-1 (Thiamin)	0.237 mg	Zinc	2.14 mg
Vitamin B-2 (Riboflavin)	0.609 mg	Copper	0.134 mg
Vitamin B-3 (Niacin)	0.586 mg	Selenium	51.8 µg
Vitamin B-5 (Pantothenic acid)	2.695 mg	Manganese	0.375 mg

EASY WAFFLES & STRAWBERRY SYRUP

SERVES	PREP TIME	COOK TIME	READY IN
4	15 min	10 min	25 min

ALLERGENS: coconut, eggs

NOTES: Nothing says weekend quite like fresh waffles. The strawberry syrup is an extra step, but well worth it!

INGREDIENTS

- 8 eggs, room temperature
- 2 Tbsp coconut oil, melted*
- 4 tsp honey
- 6 Tbsp coconut flour
- 1 tsp baking soda
- 1 tsp cinnamon

Strawberry Syrup:

- 20 large frozen strawberries
- 1/4 cup honey

*Coconut oil should be barely melted, not hot. Combining hot oil with the eggs will scramble the eggs.

DIRECTIONS

1. Preheat your waffle griddle. Whisk together the eggs. Add in the melted coconut oil and honey, whisk thoroughly. Add in the flour, baking soda, and cinnamon. Whisk together until smooth. Pour 1/4 cup of batter onto the hot griddle and cook until golden or waffle iron suggests they are done. Makes 4 large waffles.
2. For the syrup, place the frozen strawberries in a small saucepan over medium heat. Cook, stirring occasionally until strawberries become warm and soft. Transfer to a blender and puree until smooth. (Optional step.) Place the blended strawberries in a fine mesh strainer over your pan, and press the mixture with the back end of a spoon until juices drip into the pan and only pulp and seeds remain in the strainer.
3. Add honey to the pureed strawberries in the pot and warm the mixture over medium heat. Drizzle over the waffles and enjoy!

Foods Four Thought Diet

Very Berry Smoothie

Serving Size: 1 Serving

Nutrient	Quantity	Nutrient	Quantity	Nutrient	Quantity
Calories	385 kcal	Vitamin B-3	0.742 mg	Phosphorus	242 mg
Carbohydrates	55.96 g	Vitamin B-5	0.49 mg	Iron	1.8 mg
Fiber	1 g	Vitamin B-6	0.245 mg	Potassium	741 mg
Protein	8.85 g	Vitamin B-12	0.4 µg	Sodium	162 mg
Vitamin C	51.5 mg	Vitamin A	3270 IU	Zinc	0.96 mg
Folate	92 µg	Vitamin K	145.6 µg	Copper	0.122 mg
Vitamin B-1	0.178 mg	Calcium	286 mg	Selenium	6 µg
Vitamin B-2	0.522 mg	Magnesium	61 mg	Manganese	0.3 mg

Green Machine Smoothie

Serving Size: 1 Serving

Nutrient	Quantity	Nutrient	Quantity	Nutrient	Quantity
Calories	286 kcal	Vitamin B-3	1.045 mg	Phosphorus	93 mg
Carbohydrates	49.84 g	Vitamin B-5	0.639 mg	Iron	1.56 mg
Fiber	2.6 g	Vitamin B-6	0.281 mg	Potassium	611 mg
Protein	4.19 g	Vitamin B-12	0.27 µg	Sodium	55 mg
Vitamin C	61.6 mg	Vitamin A	3007 IU	Zinc	0.63 mg
Folate	100 µg	Vitamin K	146.1 µg	Copper	0.247 mg
Vitamin B-1	0.25 mg	Calcium	125 mg	Selenium	2.8 µg
Vitamin B-2	0.251 mg	Magnesium	58 mg	Manganese	1.806 mg

Orange You Glad Smoothie

Serving Size: 1 Serving

Nutrient	Quantity	Nutrient	Quantity	Nutrient	Quantity
Calories	256 kcal	Vitamin B-3	1.445 mg	Phosphorus	109 mg
Carbohydrates	43.96 g	Vitamin B-5	0.912 mg	Iron	0.57 mg
Fiber	5.8 g	Vitamin B-6	0.422 mg	Potassium	669 mg
Protein	4.29 g	Vitamin B-12	0.27 µg	Sodium	48 mg
Vitamin C	94 mg	Vitamin A	5094 IU	Zinc	0.54 mg
Folate	70 µg	Vitamin K	4.2 µg	Copper	0.169 mg
Vitamin B-1	0.204 mg	Calcium	148 mg	Selenium	3.1 µg
Vitamin B-2	0.242 mg	Magnesium	47 mg	Manganese	0.769 mg

VERY BERRY SMOOTHIE

- 2 cups frozen mixed berries
- 1 cup of orange juice
- 2 cups (handfuls) baby spinach
- 1/2 cup almond milk
- 1 Tbsp coconut oil

In a powerful blender, puree until smooth.
Serves 2

GREEN MACHINE SMOOTHIE

- 10 oz. frozen pineapple
- 1 cup of orange juice
- 2 cups (handfuls) baby spinach
- 1/2 cup coconut milk
- 1 Tbsp coconut oil

In a powerful blender, puree until smooth.
Serves 2

ORANGE YOU GLAD SMOOTHIE

- 1 frozen banana
- 1/2 cup of baby carrots
- 2 oranges
- 2 pineapple spears
- 1/2 cup coconut milk
- 1 Tbsp coconut oil

In a powerful blender, puree until smooth.
Serves 2

LUNCH & SNACKS

Energy Bites, 137

Homemade Applesauce, 139

Grain-Free Granola, 141

Candied Pecans, 143

Garlic Croutons, 145

No-Cornbread, 147

Energy Bites

NUTRITION INFORMATION

Serving Size: 1 Serving

Nutrient	Quantity	Nutrient	Quantity
Calories	276 kcal	Vitamin B-6	0.13 mg
Carbohydrates	59.09 g	Vitamin B-12 (Cobalamin)	0.03 µg
Fiber	6.2 g	Vitamin A	192 IU
Sugars	50.2 g	Vitamin E	0.25 mg
Starch	0 g	Vitamin D	4 IU
Total Fat	6.3 g	Vitamin K	2.5 µg
Omega 3	0.024 g	Calcium	45 mg
Omega 6	0.184 g	Magnesium	39 mg
Monounsaturated Fat	1.599 g	Phosphorus	56 mg
Protein	2.19 g	Iron	0.87 mg
Vitamin C	1 mg	Potassium	552 mg
Folate	15 µg	Sodium	119 mg
Vitamin B-1 (Thiamin)	0.048 mg	Zinc	0.28 mg
Vitamin B-2 (Riboflavin)	0.076 mg	Copper	0.164 mg
Vitamin B-3 (Niacin)	0.949 mg	Selenium	2.7 µg
Vitamin B-5 (Pantothenic acid)	0.458 mg	Manganese	0.293 mg

ENERGY BITES

SERVES	PREP TIME	COOK TIME	READY IN
4	15 min	0 min	15 min

ALLERGENS: almonds, coconut   **Vegan Adaptable**

NOTES: These raw treats are packed with nutrition and energy. Keep them on hand for lunchboxes or when hunger strikes.

INGREDIENTS

- 10 oz dates, pitted
- 1/2 cup almonds, slivered
- 1/2 cup shredded coconut
- 2 Tbsp almond butter
- 1 Tbsp almond milk
- 1 Tbsp honey
- 1/2 tsp cinnamon
- dash of salt

*Feel free to experiment by adding different elements such as seeds or cacao.

Makes 12 bites

DIRECTIONS

1. Add all ingredients to a food processor. Blend until the mixture starts to clump together and no large date pieces remain.
2. Shape into 1-inch balls. Roll in shredded coconut or coconut sugar if desired.
3. Refrigerate in an airtight container until ready to eat.

Homemade Applesauce

NUTRITION INFORMATION

Serving Size: 1 Serving

Nutrient	Quantity	Nutrient	Quantity
Calories	225 kcal	Vitamin B-6	0.155 mg
Carbohydrates	59.97 g	Vitamin B-12 (Cobalamin)	0 µg
Fiber	9.3 g	Vitamin A	201 IU
Sugars	46.5 g	Vitamin E	0.68 mg
Starch	0.18 g	Vitamin D	0 IU
Total Fat	0.66 g	Vitamin K	8.4 µg
Omega 3	0.033 g	Calcium	36 mg
Omega 6	0.155 g	Magnesium	20 mg
Monounsaturated Fat	0.03 g	Phosphorus	42 mg
Protein	1.04 g	Iron	0.61 mg
Vitamin C	17.3 mg	Potassium	402 mg
Folate	11 µg	Sodium	5 mg
Vitamin B-1 (Thiamin)	0.063 mg	Zinc	0.19 mg
Vitamin B-2 (Riboflavin)	0.1 mg	Copper	0.108 mg
Vitamin B-3 (Niacin)	0.364 mg	Selenium	0.1 µg
Vitamin B-5 (Pantothenic acid)	0.234 mg	Manganese	0.342 mg

HOMEMADE APPLESAUCE

SERVES	PREP TIME	COOK TIME	READY IN
4	10 min	18 min	28 min

ALLERGENS: N/A **Vegan Adaptable**

NOTES: There's nothing quite like the taste and comfort of homemade applesauce. Plus, your household will thank you too for the exquisite aroma this recipe provides.

INGREDIENTS

- 8 apples, medium-sized (Honeycrisp, Gala, or Fuji are favorites)
- 1/3 cup water (or apple juice and omit the honey)
- 2 Tbsp honey
- 1 1/2 tsp cinnamon
- 1/2 tsp pumpkin pie spice
- 1 tsp lime or lemon juice

DIRECTIONS

1. Peel, core, and chop the apples. In a large pot, combine the apples, water, honey, and spices. Cover and bring to a simmer over medium heat. Continue to simmer for 18 minutes, stirring occasionally.
2. Remove the pot from the heat. Add the apple mixture and lemon juice to a blender or food processor.
3. Enjoy warm or chilled. Store leftover applesauce in an airtight glass container. It will keep in the refrigerator for one week, or freeze and thaw at a later date.

Grain-Free Granola

NUTRITION INFORMATION

Serving Size: 1 Serving

Nutrient	Quantity	Nutrient	Quantity
Calories	316 kcal	Vitamin B-6	0.126 mg
Carbohydrates	16.72 g	Vitamin B-12 (Cobalamin)	0 μg
Fiber	3.4 g	Vitamin A	17 IU
Sugars	12.71 g	Vitamin E	0.46 mg
Starch	0.07 g	Vitamin D	0 IU
Total Fat	28.09 g	Vitamin K	0.9 μg
Omega 3	1.054 g	Calcium	34 mg
Omega 6	8.866 g	Magnesium	68 mg
Monounsaturated Fat	8.63 g	Phosphorus	136 mg
Protein	4.78 g	Iron	1.35 mg
Vitamin C	0.7 mg	Potassium	178 mg
Folate	24 μg	Sodium	94 mg
Vitamin B-1 (Thiamin)	0.186 mg	Zinc	1.56 mg
Vitamin B-2 (Riboflavin)	0.055 mg	Copper	0.453 mg
Vitamin B-3 (Niacin)	0.842 mg	Selenium	4.5 μg
Vitamin B-5 (Pantothenic acid)	0.209 mg	Manganese	1.154 mg

GRAIN-FREE GRANOLA

SERVES	PREP TIME	COOK TIME	READY IN
8	15 min	15 min	30 min

ALLERGENS: almonds, coconut, pecans, sesame, walnuts
Vegan Adaptable

NOTES: This recipe is great because you can add any kind of nuts, seeds, or dried fruits that you fancy. . . or just need to get out of your pantry.

INGREDIENTS

- 1 cup slivered almonds
- 1 cup chopped pecans
- 1 cup chopped walnuts
- 1/2 cup sesame seeds
- 1/2 cup shredded coconut
- 1/2 cup raisins (or other dried fruit)
- 1/3 cup honey
- 1/4 cup coconut oil
- 1/2 Tbsp cinnamon
- 1/4 tsp salt

DIRECTIONS

1. Preheat the oven to 325 °F. Line a cookie sheet with parchment paper.
2. Combine all of the nuts, seeds, dried fruit, and shredded coconut in a medium glass bowl. In a small saucepan melt oil over medium-low heat. Add honey and cinnamon and stir until combined. Pour over the nut mixture. Dump the entire mixture onto the prepared cookie sheet. Bake for 10–15 minutes or until golden brown.
3. Store in an air-tight container.

Candied Pecans

NUTRITION INFORMATION

Serving Size: 1 Serving

Nutrient	Quantity	Nutrient	Quantity
Calories	296 kcal	Vitamin B-6	0.08 mg
Carbohydrates	11.9 g	Vitamin B-12 (Cobalamin)	0 µg
Fiber	3.8 g	Vitamin A	22 IU
Sugars	7.95 g	Vitamin E	0.53 mg
Starch	0.17 g	Vitamin D	0 IU
Total Fat	28.42 g	Vitamin K	1.4 µg
Omega 3	0.364 g	Calcium	30 mg
Omega 6	7.686 g	Magnesium	45 mg
Monounsaturated Fat	15.247 g	Phosphorus	103 mg
Protein	3.44 g	Iron	1 mg
Vitamin C	0.5 mg	Potassium	158 mg
Folate	8 µg	Sodium	73 mg
Vitamin B-1 (Thiamin)	0.245 mg	Zinc	1.71 mg
Vitamin B-2 (Riboflavin)	0.051 mg	Copper	0.449 mg
Vitamin B-3 (Niacin)	0.447 mg	Selenium	1.5 µg
Vitamin B-5 (Pantothenic acid)	0.327 mg	Manganese	1.734 mg

CANDIED PECANS

SERVES	PREP TIME	COOK TIME	READY IN
8	10 min	1 hr	1 hr 10 min

ALLERGENS: coconut, pecans   **Vegan Adaptable**

NOTES: The flavor of these crunchy delights is perfect and without any refined sugar. Pecans are also a great source of energy. Munch at your leisure, bag them up as gifts, or use them in a salad or over tasty fruit and cream.

INGREDIENTS

- 3 cups pecans
- 3 Tbsp honey
- 1 Tbsp coconut oil, melted
- 1 tsp cinnamon
- 1/4 tsp salt

DIRECTIONS

1. Preheat your oven to 250 °F. Line a baking sheet with parchment paper.
2. Place the pecans in a medium-size bowl. In a separate small bowl, whisk together the honey, oil, cinnamon, and salt until combined.
3. Pour the wet mixture into the pecan bowl and toss until evenly coated.
4. Pour the pecans onto the prepared baking sheet and spread out into an even layer.
5. Bake in the preheated oven for 1 hour, tossing every 20 minutes.
6. Cool, and store in an airtight container.

Garlic Croutons

NUTRITION INFORMATION

Serving Size: 1 Serving

Nutrient	Quantity	Nutrient	Quantity
Calories	164 kcal	Vitamin B-6	0.154 mg
Carbohydrates	2.59 g	Vitamin B-12 (Cobalamin)	2.54 µg
Fiber	0.5 g	Vitamin A	681 IU
Sugars	1.3 g	Vitamin E	0.93 mg
Starch	0 g	Vitamin D	38 IU
Total Fat	14.2 g	Vitamin K	1.3 µg
Omega 3	0.073 g	Calcium	42 mg
Omega 6	0.754 g	Magnesium	16 mg
Monounsaturated Fat	5.041 g	Phosphorus	114 mg
Protein	6.42 g	Iron	1.99 mg
Vitamin C	5.7 mg	Potassium	192 mg
Folate	39 µg	Sodium	368 mg
Vitamin B-1 (Thiamin)	0.087 mg	Zinc	0.73 mg
Vitamin B-2 (Riboflavin)	0.213 mg	Copper	0.049 mg
Vitamin B-3 (Niacin)	0.167 mg	Selenium	17.6 µg
Vitamin B-5 (Pantothenic acid)	0.906 mg	Manganese	0.089 mg

GARLIC CROUTONS

SERVES	PREP TIME	COOK TIME	READY IN
6	15 min	40 min	55 min

ALLERGENS: coconut, eggs

NOTES: Switch up your salad game with some delicious homemade croutons. These are of course grain-free and bursting with garlic goodness.

INGREDIENTS

- 4 eggs
- 1/4 cup ghee
- 3 cloves garlic, minced
- 2/3 cups coconut flour
- 1/2 tsp salt
- 1/2 tsp paprika
- 1/2 tsp Italian seasoning
- 1/4 tsp pepper

DIRECTIONS

1. Preheat your oven to 350 °F. Line a baking sheet with parchment paper.
2. Combine the eggs, ghee, and garlic with an electric mixer. Add in the coconut flour and spices. Mix until combined. The dough will be slightly crumbly.
3. Drop the dough onto the parchment paper and form into a square or rectangle that is 1/2 inch thick. I used a large rubber spatula to do this. Sprinkle with additional sea salt.
4. Bake in the preheated oven for 20 minutes.
5. Remove from the oven and slice into 1/2 inch cubes. Separate and spread around the baking sheet. Bake for another 15–20 minutes depending on your desired crunch.

No-Cornbread

NUTRITION INFORMATION

Serving Size: 1 Serving

Nutrient	Quantity	Nutrient	Quantity
Calories	241 kcal	Vitamin B-6	0.098 mg
Carbohydrates	12.25 g	Vitamin B-12 (Cobalamin)	1.89 µg
Fiber	0.3 g	Vitamin A	236 IU
Sugars	11.78 g	Vitamin E	0.48 mg
Starch	0 g	Vitamin D	24 IU
Total Fat	20.19 g	Vitamin K	0.2 µg
Omega 3	0.032 g	Calcium	29 mg
Omega 6	0.673 g	Magnesium	12 mg
Monounsaturated Fat	3.174 g	Phosphorus	82 mg
Protein	4.69 g	Iron	1.48 mg
Vitamin C	0.6 mg	Potassium	141 mg
Folate	29 µg	Sodium	221 mg
Vitamin B-1 (Thiamin)	0.061 mg	Zinc	0.55 mg
Vitamin B-2 (Riboflavin)	0.159 mg	Copper	0.036 mg
Vitamin B-3 (Niacin)	0.104 mg	Selenium	13.1 µg
Vitamin B-5 (Pantothenic acid)	0.67 mg	Manganese	0.058 mg

NO-CORNBREAD

SERVES	PREP TIME	COOK TIME	READY IN
8	12 min	18 min	30 min

ALLERGENS: coconut, eggs

NOTES: This is about as close to cornbread as you're going to get while eliminating corn. This remaster of a traditional favorite is very tasty and makes a perfect side to any dinner or steaming bowl of chili.

INGREDIENTS

- 4 eggs
- 1/2 cup coconut oil, melted*
- 1/4 cup honey
- 3/4 cup coconut flour
- 1/2 tsp salt
- 1 tsp baking soda
- 1 tsp apple cider vinegar

Drizzle

- 1 Tbsp coconut oil, melted (or ghee)
- 1 Tbsp honey

*Coconut oil should be barely melted, not hot. Combining hot oil with the eggs will scramble the eggs.

DIRECTIONS

1. Preheat the oven to 350 °F. Grease an 8 x 8 glass baking dish.
2. In a medium-sized bowl, with an electric mixer beat together the eggs, oil, and honey. Pour in the coconut flour and salt, and beat until combined. Add in the baking soda and vinegar and mix until just combined, do not over-mix. Spread and press the batter into the prepared baking dish. Bake in the preheated oven for 18 minutes or until golden around the edges of the pan.
3. Meanwhile, whisk together the coconut oil and honey. Drizzle over the warm no-cornbread and spread with the backside of a spoon.

DINNER

Thai Tahini Salad, 151

Spiced Cream Soup, 153

Amazing Vinaigrette, 155

Creamy Asparagus Soup, 157

Lime Cilantro Salad, 159

Vegetable Chili, 161

Poppy Seed Salad, 163

Pumpkin Soup, 165

Curried Salad, 167

Creamy Curried Soup, 169

Honey Mustard Salad, 171

Easy Creamy Vegetable Soup, 173

Strawberry Spinach Salad, 175

Creamy Red Pepper Soup, 177

Thai Tahini Salad

NUTRITION INFORMATION

Serving Size: 1 Serving

Nutrient	Quantity	Nutrient	Quantity
Calories	230 kcal	Vitamin B-6	0.173 mg
Carbohydrates	12.05 g	Vitamin B-12 (Cobalamin)	0.01 µg
Fiber	1.6 g	Vitamin A	5541 IU
Sugars	8.45 g	Vitamin E	4.2 mg
Starch	0 g	Vitamin D	0 IU
Total Fat	20.25 g	Vitamin K	289.8 µg
Omega 3	0.359 g	Calcium	66 mg
Omega 6	2.834 g	Magnesium	51 mg
Monounsaturated Fat	13.518 g	Phosphorus	40 mg
Protein	2.2 g	Iron	1.91 mg
Vitamin C	45.9 mg	Potassium	404 mg
Folate	115 µg	Sodium	472 mg
Vitamin B-1 (Thiamin)	0.063 mg	Zinc	0.4 mg
Vitamin B-2 (Riboflavin)	0.129 mg	Copper	0.109 mg
Vitamin B-3 (Niacin)	0.568 mg	Selenium	1.2 µg
Vitamin B-5 (Pantothenic acid)	0.074 mg	Manganese	0.6 mg

THAI TAHINI SALAD

SERVES	PREP TIME	COOK TIME	READY IN
4	15 min	0 min	15 min

ALLERGENS: coconut, sesame   **Vegan Adaptable**

NOTES: I just can't go without this dressing, it is so good! I often use it to drizzle over Asian Lettuce Wraps, a fresh spinach salad, or just skip all of that and eat it by the spoonful as I hover over the kitchen counter.

INGREDIENTS

Dressing:
- 1/3 cup olive oil
- 1/4 cup creamy tahini
- 2 Tbsp apple cider vinegar
- 1/2 lime, juiced
- 1 1/2 Tbsp coconut aminos
- 1 1/2 Tbsp honey
- 2 cloves garlic
- 1 tsp ginger, dried & ground
- 1/2 tsp salt
- 1/4 cup cilantro
- Pepper to taste

Salad:
- 1/2 lb. baby spinach or leaf lettuce

DIRECTIONS

1. Place all ingredients into a powerful blender and puree until completely smooth. Serve over fresh greens and your choice of fresh toppings.

Topping ideas: bell pepper, olives, chives, shredded carrots, avocado, cashew pieces

*Can be substituted for cashew butter.

Spiced Cream Soup

NUTRITION INFORMATION

Serving Size: 1 Serving

Nutrient	Quantity	Nutrient	Quantity
Calories	246 kcal	Vitamin B-6	0.287 mg
Carbohydrates	20.12 g	Vitamin B-12 (Cobalamin)	0 µg
Fiber	5.6 g	Vitamin A	19457 IU
Sugars	6.62 g	Vitamin E	2.05 mg
Starch	1.62 g	Vitamin D	0 IU
Total Fat	17.77 g	Vitamin K	34.1 µg
Omega 3	0.156 g	Calcium	168 mg
Omega 6	5.606 g	Magnesium	46 mg
Monounsaturated Fat	8.967 g	Phosphorus	200 mg
Protein	5.08 g	Iron	2.86 mg
Vitamin C	19.2 mg	Potassium	525 mg
Folate	57 µg	Sodium	1275 mg
Vitamin B-1 (Thiamin)	0.341 mg	Zinc	1.28 mg
Vitamin B-2 (Riboflavin)	0.175 mg	Copper	0.435 mg
Vitamin B-3 (Niacin)	2.357 mg	Selenium	7.6 µg
Vitamin B-5 (Pantothenic acid)	0.513 mg	Manganese	0.664 mg

SPICED CREAM SOUP

SERVES	PREP TIME	COOK TIME	READY IN
4	15 min	25 min	40 min

ALLERGENS: sesame   **Vegan**

NOTES: Everyone will enjoy the warm and robust flavor of this comforting creamy soup. Feel free to double the recipe and freeze half for future use.

INGREDIENTS

- 2 Tbsp olive oil
- 1 large leek stalk, sliced*
- 4 garlic cloves, minced
- 2 tsp salt
- 1/4 tsp pepper
- 1/4 tsp turmeric
- 1/4 tsp thyme
- 16 oz carrots, chopped
- 4 cups water (or broth)
- 1/2 lime, juiced
- 1/3 cup tahini
- 1/3 cup cilantro

*You can substitute the leak for a large yellow onion.

DIRECTIONS

1. In a large pot, over medium heat, add the olive oil and leek. Sauté until translucent, about 4 minutes. Add the garlic and spices. Sauté for another 1 minute.
2. Add the carrots and water. Stir and cover. Allow to simmer for 20 minutes, or until carrots are tender.
3. Transfer to a powerful blender. Add in the lime, tahini, and cilantro. Blend until smooth.
4. Serve with the Garlic Crouton recipe or additional garnish if desired.

Amazing Vinaigrette Salad

NUTRITION INFORMATION

Serving Size: 1 Serving

Nutrient	Quantity	Nutrient	Quantity
Calories	272 kcal	Vitamin B-6	0.171 mg
Carbohydrates	6.2 g	Vitamin B-12 (Cobalamin)	0 µg
Fiber	1.8 g	Vitamin A	7111 IU
Sugars	2.99 g	Vitamin E	5.42 mg
Starch	0 g	Vitamin D	0 IU
Total Fat	27.31 g	Vitamin K	381.6 µg
Omega 3	0.31 g	Calcium	81 mg
Omega 6	2.641 g	Magnesium	62 mg
Monounsaturated Fat	19.707 g	Phosphorus	42 mg
Protein	2.35 g	Iron	2.33 mg
Vitamin C	26.3 mg	Potassium	447 mg
Folate	147 µg	Sodium	257 mg
Vitamin B-1 (Thiamin)	0.064 mg	Zinc	0.44 mg
Vitamin B-2 (Riboflavin)	0.147 mg	Copper	0.109 mg
Vitamin B-3 (Niacin)	0.577 mg	Selenium	1 µg
Vitamin B-5 (Pantothenic acid)	0.06 mg	Manganese	0.723 mg

AMAZING VINAIGRETTE SALAD

SERVES	PREP TIME	COOK TIME	READY IN
6	15 min	0 min	15 min

ALLERGENS: N/A   **Vegan Adaptable**

NOTES: This is hands down, a favorite dressing in our home. The final result is perfectly creamy and full of exciting zesty flavor.

INGREDIENTS

- 3/4 cup olive oil (light tasting)
- 1/4 cup balsamic vinegar
- 3 cloves garlic
- 1/2 tsp salt
- 1/4 tsp pepper
- 1 tsp honey
- 1 lb. spinach or preferred greens

DIRECTIONS

1. Place all ingredients in a powerful blender. Puree until smooth and thoroughly combined.
2. Drizzle over greens and garnish with desired toppings.

Topping ideas: slivered almonds, olives, chives, avocado

Creamy Asparagus Soup

NUTRITION INFORMATION

Serving Size: 1 Serving

Nutrient	Quantity	Nutrient	Quantity
Calories	106 kcal	Vitamin B-6	0.35 mg
Carbohydrates	16.06 g	Vitamin B-12 (Cobalamin)	0 µg
Fiber	5.6 g	Vitamin A	1749 IU
Sugars	8.58 g	Vitamin E	2.6 mg
Starch	0 g	Vitamin D	0 IU
Total Fat	3.76 g	Vitamin K	95.1 µg
Omega 3	0.023 g	Calcium	85 mg
Omega 6	0.16 g	Magnesium	42 mg
Monounsaturated Fat	0.198 g	Phosphorus	145 mg
Protein	5.85 g	Iron	5.15 mg
Vitamin C	24.2 mg	Potassium	575 mg
Folate	138 µg	Sodium	886 mg
Vitamin B-1 (Thiamin)	0.365 mg	Zinc	1.37 mg
Vitamin B-2 (Riboflavin)	0.341 mg	Copper	0.494 mg
Vitamin B-3 (Niacin)	2.371 mg	Selenium	6 µg
Vitamin B-5 (Pantothenic acid)	0.718 mg	Manganese	0.468 mg

CREAMY ASPARAGUS SOUP

SERVES	PREP TIME	COOK TIME	READY IN
4	10 min	22 min	32 min

ALLERGENS: coconut   **Vegan**

NOTES: There is something magical about the flavor of this soup. It's deep yet refreshing. Even if you're not big on asparagus, you and your family are sure to enjoy this nutrient-rich dish.

INGREDIENTS

- 1 Tbsp coconut oil
- 1 large sweet onion, chopped
- 2 lbs. asparagus, 2 inches of base removed
- 3 large garlic cloves, chopped
- 1 1/2 cups water*
- 1 1/2 tsp sea salt
- 1/4 tsp pepper

*If you have broth available, especially if it is homemade, feel free to use it. You may however need to adjust the amount of salt in the recipe.

DIRECTIONS

1. Place the oil in a large pot over medium-high heat. Add the onion and sauté for 3 minutes.
2. Cut the asparagus spears in half and place them in the pot along with the garlic. Sauté for 4 more minutes or until the vegetables are barely tender and the onions are translucent.
3. Add the water, salt, and pepper. Cover the pot and allow to simmer for 15 minutes.
4. Transfer to a powerful blender and puree until smooth.
5. Freeze or refrigerate any leftovers.

Lime Cilantro Salad

NUTRITION INFORMATION

Serving Size: 1 Serving

Nutrient	Quantity	Nutrient	Quantity
Calories	277 kcal	Vitamin B-6	0.37 mg
Carbohydrates	11.6 g	Vitamin B-12 (Cobalamin)	0 µg
Fiber	4.9 g	Vitamin A	6472 IU
Sugars	1.84 g	Vitamin E	3.92 mg
Starch	0.06 g	Vitamin D	0 IU
Total Fat	25.72 g	Vitamin K	147.1 µg
Omega 3	0.194 g	Calcium	49 mg
Omega 6	2.622 g	Magnesium	36 mg
Monounsaturated Fat	18.058 g	Phosphorus	72 mg
Protein	2.99 g	Iron	1.96 mg
Vitamin C	119.5 mg	Potassium	575 mg
Folate	87 µg	Sodium	620 mg
Vitamin B-1 (Thiamin)	0.115 mg	Zinc	0.65 mg
Vitamin B-2 (Riboflavin)	0.156 mg	Copper	0.201 mg
Vitamin B-3 (Niacin)	1.771 mg	Selenium	1.8 µg
Vitamin B-5 (Pantothenic acid)	0.943 mg	Manganese	0.38 mg

LIME CILANTRO SALAD

SERVES	PREP TIME	COOK TIME	READY IN
4	15 min	0 min	15 min

ALLERGENS: N/A   **Vegan**

NOTES: The lime and apple cider gives this dressing an irresistible zing. Garnish with fresh crunchy bell peppers for an exciting crunch along with anything else you can dream up for this exciting salad.

INGREDIENTS

- 1 red bell pepper, diced
- 1 yellow bell pepper, diced
- 1/3 cup green onions, diced
- 1 head red leaf lettuce, chopped
- avocado (optional garnish)
- olives (optional garnish)

Dressing

- 1/3 cup olive oil
- 3 Tbsp apple cider vinegar
- 1/2 lime, juiced
- 1 garlic clove, chopped
- 1/2 tsp cumin
- 1 tsp salt
- 1/4 tsp pepper
- 1/2 cup cilantro, chopped

DIRECTIONS

1. Place the chopped red leaf lettuce in a large salad bowl and drain off any excess water. Put the bell peppers in a separate medium bowl. Set both aside in the refrigerator.
2. Place the dressing ingredients into a powerful blender, preferably with a small jar attachment. Blend until completely smooth.
3. Add two tablespoons of the dressing to the bell peppers and toss.
4. Pour the remaining dressing over the lettuce and toss with the bell peppers. Garnish with sliced olives and avocado or any other desired FFT approved veggies or nuts.

Vegetable Chili

NUTRITION INFORMATION

Serving Size: 1 Serving

Nutrient	Quantity	Nutrient	Quantity
Calories	86 kcal	Vitamin B-6	0.293 mg
Carbohydrates	14.57 g	Vitamin B-12 (Cobalamin)	0 µg
Fiber	4.2 g	Vitamin A	11500 IU
Sugars	7.59 g	Vitamin E	2.01 mg
Starch	0 g	Vitamin D	0 IU
Total Fat	2.92 g	Vitamin K	18.2 µg
Omega 3	0.032 g	Calcium	71 mg
Omega 6	0.428 g	Magnesium	26 mg
Monounsaturated Fat	1.789 g	Phosphorus	57 mg
Protein	1.85 g	Iron	1.82 mg
Vitamin C	34.5 mg	Potassium	394 mg
Folate	41 µg	Sodium	995 mg
Vitamin B-1 (Thiamin)	0.072 mg	Zinc	0.41 mg
Vitamin B-2 (Riboflavin)	0.085 mg	Copper	0.178 mg
Vitamin B-3 (Niacin)	1.029 mg	Selenium	1.8 µg
Vitamin B-5 (Pantothenic acid)	0.434 mg	Manganese	0.284 mg

VEGETABLE CHILI

SERVES	PREP TIME	COOK TIME	READY IN
6	15 min	55 min	1 hr 10 min

ALLERGENS: N/A **Vegan**

NOTES: This hearty vegetable chili is savory and satisfying. Feel free to double up the recipe as this is one of those blessed dishes that get better as they sit in the refrigerator.

INGREDIENTS

- 1 Tbsp olive oil, divided
- 16 oz bag baby carrots, sliced
- 1 large sweet onion, diced
- 1 red bell pepper, diced
- 1 green bell pepper, diced
- 3 stalks celery, sliced
- 3 cloves garlic, minced
- 2 Tbsp chili powder
- 2 tsp sea salt
- 2 tsp Italian seasoning
- 1 tsp cumin
- 3 1/2 cups water*
- 1/4 cup cilantro, chopped

DIRECTIONS

1. In a large pot heat the olive oil over medium-high heat and sauté the vegetables for 10 minutes.
2. Add the chili powder, salt, other seasonings, and water.
3. Bring to a boil, then reduce heat to low, cover, and simmer for 45 minutes.
4. Garnish with cilantro.

*If you have broth available, especially if it is homemade, feel free to use it. You may however need to adjust the amount of salt in the recipe.

Poppy Seed Salad

NUTRITION INFORMATION

Serving Size: 1 Serving

Nutrient	Quantity	Nutrient	Quantity
Calories	474 kcal	Vitamin B-6	0.205 mg
Carbohydrates	33.04 g	Vitamin B-12 (Cobalamin)	0 µg
Fiber	3 g	Vitamin A	5814 IU
Sugars	23.93 g	Vitamin E	4.31 mg
Starch	5.03 g	Vitamin D	0 IU
Total Fat	37.54 g	Vitamin K	132.9 µg
Omega 3	0.233 g	Calcium	73 mg
Omega 6	4.938 g	Magnesium	84 mg
Monounsaturated Fat	24.928 g	Phosphorus	177 mg
Protein	5.58 g	Iron	2.94 mg
Vitamin C	5.4 mg	Potassium	380 mg
Folate	37 µg	Sodium	621 mg
Vitamin B-1 (Thiamin)	0.17 mg	Zinc	1.65 mg
Vitamin B-2 (Riboflavin)	0.096 mg	Copper	0.55 mg
Vitamin B-3 (Niacin)	0.573 mg	Selenium	6.4 µg
Vitamin B-5 (Pantothenic acid)	0.352 mg	Manganese	0.758 mg

POPPY SEED SALAD

SERVES	PREP TIME	COOK TIME	READY IN
4	15 min	0 min	15 min

ALLERGENS: cashews **Vegan Adaptable**

NOTES: The flavors of this poppy seed salad are positively delicious. Experiment with different lettuces, fruit, and nuts to find your favorite combo.

INGREDIENTS

- 1 head red leaf lettuce
- 1 Honeycrisp apple, peeled, cored, and finely cubed
- 1/3 cup cashews, chopped

Dressing:
- 1/2 cup olive oil
- 1/3 cup apple cider vinegar
- 1/4 cup honey
- 1 clove garlic, chopped
- 1 Tbsp poppy seeds
- 1 tsp salt
- 1 tsp dry mustard

DIRECTIONS

1. Place the lettuce in a large salad bowl. Set aside in the refrigerator.
2. Place the dressing ingredients into a powerful blender, preferably with a small jar attachment. Blend until completely smooth.
3. Pour over the spinach and toss. Garnish with apples, cashews, and any other FFT approved veggies, fruit, or seeds.

Pumpkin Soup

NUTRITION INFORMATION

Serving Size: 1 Serving

Nutrient	Quantity	Nutrient	Quantity
Calories	207 kcal	Vitamin B-6	0.07 mg
Carbohydrates	12.18 g	Vitamin B-12 (Cobalamin)	0 µg
Fiber	2 g	Vitamin A	365 IU
Sugars	6.1 g	Vitamin E	0.46 mg
Starch	0 g	Vitamin D	0 IU
Total Fat	17.86 g	Vitamin K	29.9 µg
Omega 3	0.054 g	Calcium	25 mg
Omega 6	0.956 g	Magnesium	27 mg
Monounsaturated Fat	1.166 g	Phosphorus	65 mg
Protein	2.78 g	Iron	1.17 mg
Vitamin C	6.6 mg	Potassium	230 mg
Folate	11 µg	Sodium	396 mg
Vitamin B-1 (Thiamin)	0.03 mg	Zinc	0.93 mg
Vitamin B-2 (Riboflavin)	0.023 mg	Copper	0.201 mg
Vitamin B-3 (Niacin)	0.414 mg	Selenium	0.4 µg
Vitamin B-5 (Pantothenic acid)	0.168 mg	Manganese	0.612 mg

PUMPKIN SOUP

SERVES	PREP TIME	COOK TIME	READY IN
6	15 min	18 min	33 min

ALLERGENS: coconut   **Vegan Adaptable**

NOTES: This pumpkin soup is so warm, savory, and soothing. Get all the benefits of pumpkin, including potassium and vitamin A, in one comforting bowl.

INGREDIENTS

- 1 Tbsp coconut oil
- 1/2 yellow onion, chopped
- 3 cloves garlic, chopped
- 1–14 oz can pumpkin puree
- 2 cups water*
- 1 cup coconut cream**
- 2 Tbsp honey
- 1 tsp salt

*If you have broth available, especially if it is homemade, feel free to use it. You may however need to adjust the amount of salt in the recipe.

**I generally get coconut cream by refrigerating 1 can of coconut milk and removing the solidified cream at the top. Save remaining milk for another use.

DIRECTIONS

1. In a large pot, melt the coconut oil over medium-high heat. Sauté the onion and garlic for 3 minutes. Add in the pumpkin puree, and water.
2. Reduce the temperature to medium-low and allow to simmer for 15 minutes.
3. Transfer to a powerful blender. Add in the coconut milk, honey, and salt. Blend until completely smooth.
4. Garnish with chives, nuts, seeds, or croutons.

Curried Salad

NUTRITION INFORMATION

Serving Size: 1 Serving

Nutrient	Quantity	Nutrient	Quantity
Calories	194 kcal	Vitamin B-6	0.085 mg
Carbohydrates	12.54 g	Vitamin B-12 (Cobalamin)	0 µg
Fiber	2.3 g	Vitamin A	2524 IU
Sugars	9.9 g	Vitamin E	2.51 mg
Starch	0.04 g	Vitamin D	0 IU
Total Fat	16.14 g	Vitamin K	134.2 µg
Omega 3	0.201 g	Calcium	45 mg
Omega 6	2.324 g	Magnesium	32 mg
Monounsaturated Fat	10.982 g	Phosphorus	37 mg
Protein	1.67 g	Iron	1.12 mg
Vitamin C	18.3 mg	Potassium	233 mg
Folate	55 µg	Sodium	234 mg
Vitamin B-1 (Thiamin)	0.091 mg	Zinc	0.46 mg
Vitamin B-2 (Riboflavin)	0.079 mg	Copper	0.127 mg
Vitamin B-3 (Niacin)	0.397 mg	Selenium	1.3 µg
Vitamin B-5 (Pantothenic acid)	0.155 mg	Manganese	0.593 mg

CURRIED SALAD

SERVES	PREP TIME	COOK TIME	READY IN
6	15 min	0 min	15 min

ALLERGENS: pecans   **Vegan Adaptable**

NOTES: The flavors of this salad are so pleasant, delicious, and satisfying. Play around with different fruits, vegetables, nuts, or seeds to adorn this uplifting salad.

INGREDIENTS

- 1/3 lb baby spinach
- 2 mandarin oranges, segmented
- 1/2 cup fresh blueberries
- 1/4 cup green onion, chopped
- 1/3 cup candied pecans

Dressing:
- 1/3 cup olive oil
- 1/3 cup apple cider vinegar
- 1 Tbsp honey
- 2 tsp dijon mustard
- 1 tsp curry powder
- 1/2 tsp salt

DIRECTIONS

1. In a small bowl whisk together the dressing ingredients.
2. Place your spinach in a large salad bowl. Pour the dressing over the salad and toss.
3. Garnish with mandarin orange slices, blueberries, green onion, and candied pecans.

Creamy Curry Soup

NUTRITION INFORMATION

Serving Size: 1 Serving

Nutrient	Quantity	Nutrient	Quantity
Calories	78 kcal	Vitamin B-6	0.165 mg
Carbohydrates	7.95 g	Vitamin B-12 (Cobalamin)	0.12 µg
Fiber	2.5 g	Vitamin A	6898 IU
Sugars	3.26 g	Vitamin E	0.76 mg
Starch	0.59 g	Vitamin D	0 IU
Total Fat	3.92 g	Vitamin K	14 µg
Omega 3	0.349 g	Calcium	66 mg
Omega 6	0.625g	Magnesium	15 mg
Monounsaturated Fat	0.555 g	Phosphorus	74 mg
Protein	3.74 g	Iron	0.72 mg
Vitamin C	19.7 mg	Potassium	368 mg
Folate	33 µg	Sodium	719 mg
Vitamin B-1 (Thiamin)	0.053 mg	Zinc	0.38 mg
Vitamin B-2 (Riboflavin)	0.088 mg	Copper	0.109 mg
Vitamin B-3 (Niacin)	2.287 mg	Selenium	1.5 µg
Vitamin B-5 (Pantothenic acid)	0.37 mg	Manganese	0.202 mg

CREAMY CURRY SOUP

SERVES	PREP TIME	COOK TIME	READY IN
8	20 min	25 min	40 min

ALLERGENS: coconut   **Vegan**

NOTES: This Thai soup will put some pep in your step and is great any time of the year. This recipe makes a large batch making it a perfect addition to your meal prep. Feel free to freeze half in mason jars or use it as a tasty cream sauce over veggies or poultry.

INGREDIENTS

- 1 Tbsp coconut oil
- 3 cups baby carrots, chopped
- 1 large yellow onion, chopped
- 2 cloves garlic
- 1 head cauliflower, cut into florets
- 4 cups broth*
- 1/2 lime, juiced
- 1 Tbsp curry powder
- 2 tsp ginger, dried & ground
- 1 tsp salt

*You can also use 4 cups of water and 1 tsp salt if broth is not available.

DIRECTIONS

1. In a large pot heat the oil over medium-high heat. Add the carrots, onion, and garlic to the pot and sauté for 5 minutes. Add the broth, cauliflower, lime, and spices. Cover and simmer for 20 minutes.
2. Transfer to a powerful blender in two separate batches to ensure a creamy texture. Puree until completely smooth. Serve hot and garnish with cilantro, chives, lime wedges, coconut cream or enjoy as is.
3. Refrigerate or freeze any leftovers.

Honey Mustard Salad

NUTRITION INFORMATION

Serving Size: 1 Serving

Nutrient	Quantity	Nutrient	Quantity
Calories	274 kcal	Vitamin B-6	0.159 mg
Carbohydrates	27.26 g	Vitamin B-12 (Cobalamin)	0 µg
Fiber	1.8 g	Vitamin A	6095 IU
Sugars	24.31 g	Vitamin E	2.86 mg
Starch	0.13 g	Vitamin D	0 IU
Total Fat	18.8 g	Vitamin K	127.9 µg
Omega 3	0.217 g	Calcium	45 mg
Omega 6	1.827 g	Magnesium	23 mg
Monounsaturated Fat	13.493 g	Phosphorus	51 mg
Protein	2.15 g	Iron	1.62 mg
Vitamin C	19.8 mg	Potassium	235 mg
Folate	34 µg	Sodium	540 mg
Vitamin B-1 (Thiamin)	0.095 mg	Zinc	0.39 mg
Vitamin B-2 (Riboflavin)	0.096 mg	Copper	0.064 mg
Vitamin B-3 (Niacin)	0.556 mg	Selenium	8.4 µg
Vitamin B-5 (Pantothenic acid)	0.212 mg	Manganese	0.297 mg

HONEY MUSTARD SALAD

SERVES	PREP TIME	COOK TIME	READY IN
4	15 min	0 min	15 min

ALLERGENS: almonds

NOTES: There was a time when my son would eat anything so long as there was honey mustard involved. So I'm gifting this recipe to you in hopes that it may serve you as well.

INGREDIENTS

- 1 head red leaf lettuce
- 1 red bell pepper, diced
- 1/4 cup green onions
- 1/3 cup slivered almonds

Dressing:

- 1/3 cup olive oil
- 1/3 cup yellow mustard
- 1/3 cup honey
- 1/2 tsp salt

DIRECTIONS

1. In a small bowl whisk together the dressing ingredients.
2. Place your lettuce in a large salad bowl. Pour the desired amount of dressing over the lettuce and toss. Store any leftover dressing in the fridge for later use or vegetable dip.
3. Garnish the salad with diced bell peppers, green onions, and slivered almonds.

Easy Creamy Vegetable Soup

NUTRITION INFORMATION

Serving Size: 1 Serving

Nutrient	Quantity	Nutrient	Quantity
Calories	83 kcal	Vitamin B-6	0.316 mg
Carbohydrates	11.05 g	Vitamin B-12 (Cobalamin)	0 μg
Fiber	3.9 g	Vitamin A	947 IU
Sugars	4.28 g	Vitamin E	0.82 mg
Starch	0.01 g	Vitamin D	0 IU
Total Fat	3.84 g	Vitamin K	47.6 μg
Omega 3	0.044 g	Calcium	82 mg
Omega 6	0.409 g	Magnesium	32 mg
Monounsaturated Fat	2.526 g	Phosphorus	76 mg
Protein	3.03 g	Iron	0.86 mg
Vitamin C	60.5 mg	Potassium	552 mg
Folate	91 μg	Sodium	962 mg
Vitamin B-1 (Thiamin)	0.088 mg	Zinc	0.47 mg
Vitamin B-2 (Riboflavin)	0.115 mg	Copper	0.1 mg
Vitamin B-3 (Niacin)	0.842 mg	Selenium	1.4 μg
Vitamin B-5 (Pantothenic acid)	0.929 mg	Manganese	0.328 mg

EASY CREAMY VEGETABLE SOUP

SERVES	PREP TIME	COOK TIME	READY IN
8	10 min	35 min	45 min

ALLERGENS: N/A   **Vegan**

NOTES: A delicious warm soup makes any day a little brighter. This soup hits the spot and is easy to make and store in the freezer for future meals.

INGREDIENTS

- 2 Tbsp olive oil
- 2 medium onions, chopped
- 1–16 oz bag baby carrots, halved
- 5 celery ribs, chopped
- 6 cloves garlic, chopped
- 8 cups riced cauliflower (or 2 heads)
- 6 cups of water
- 3 tsp salt
- 1 Tbsp parsley, dried
- 1 tsp basil, dried
- 1/2 tsp oregano, dried
- 1/4 tsp pepper

DIRECTIONS

1. Over medium-high heat, add the olive oil to a large pot. Sauté the onions, carrots, celery, and garlic for 5 minutes.
2. Add the cauliflower, water, herbs, and spices. Cover and simmer over low heat for 30 minutes or until the carrots are very tender.
3. Transfer half of the soup to a powerful blender. Puree until smooth. Transfer to a large glass bowl and repeat with the second half of the soup. Serve hot and enjoy.

Strawberry Spinach Salad

NUTRITION INFORMATION

Serving Size: 1 Serving

Nutrient	Quantity	Nutrient	Quantity
Calories	422 kcal	Vitamin B-6	0.131 mg
Carbohydrates	23.89 g	Vitamin B-12 (Cobalamin)	0 µg
Fiber	2.9 g	Vitamin A	3555 IU
Sugars	20.07 g	Vitamin E	4.95 mg
Starch	0.08 g	Vitamin D	0 IU
Total Fat	37.07 g	Vitamin K	198.7 µg
Omega 3	0.414 g	Calcium	56 mg
Omega 6	5.48 g	Magnesium	53 mg
Monounsaturated Fat	25.278 g	Phosphorus	68 mg
Protein	2.68 g	Iron	1.81 mg
Vitamin C	38.8 mg	Potassium	352 mg
Folate	85 µg	Sodium	323 mg
Vitamin B-1 (Thiamin)	0.13 mg	Zinc	0.93 mg
Vitamin B-2 (Riboflavin)	0.107 mg	Copper	0.243 mg
Vitamin B-3 (Niacin)	0.621 mg	Selenium	1.2 µg
Vitamin B-5 (Pantothenic acid)	0.203 mg	Manganese	1.149 mg

STRAWBERRY SPINACH SALAD

SERVES	PREP TIME	COOK TIME	READY IN
4	15 min	0 min	15 min

ALLERGENS: pecans   **Vegan Adaptable**

NOTES: A classic strawberry spinach salad recipe without the high sugar content. This salad always makes its way onto someone's birthday dinner list.

INGREDIENTS

- 1/3 lb spinach,
- 1 cup strawberries, sliced
- 1/2 candied pecans

Dressing:

- 1/2 cup olive oil
- 1/4 cup apple cider vinegar
- 1/4 cup raw honey
- 1/2 tsp salt
- 1/4 tsp cracked pepper

DIRECTIONS

1. In a small bowl whisk together the vinaigrette ingredients.
2. Place your spinach and strawberries in a large bowl. Pour the dressing over the salad and toss.
3. Garnish with candied pecans.

Creamy Red Pepper Soup

NUTRITION INFORMATION

Serving Size: 1 Serving

Nutrient	Quantity	Nutrient	Quantity
Calories	157 kcal	Vitamin B-6	0.308 mg
Carbohydrates	9.78 g	Vitamin B-12 (Cobalamin)	0.08 μg
Fiber	2.8 g	Vitamin A	4208 IU
Sugars	4.77 g	Vitamin E	2.24 mg
Starch	0.15 g	Vitamin D	0 IU
Total Fat	12.18 g	Vitamin K	8.5 μg
Omega 3	0.246 g	Calcium	42 mg
Omega 6	0.533 g	Magnesium	20 mg
Monounsaturated Fat	3.666 g	Phosphorus	80 mg
Protein	3.45 g	Iron	1.1 mg
Vitamin C	108.9 mg	Potassium	369 mg
Folate	50 μg	Sodium	1028 mg
Vitamin B-1 (Thiamin)	0.069 mg	Zinc	0.55 mg
Vitamin B-2 (Riboflavin)	0.104 mg	Copper	0.148 mg
Vitamin B-3 (Niacin)	2.14 mg	Selenium	0.9 μg
Vitamin B-5 (Pantothenic acid)	0.364 mg	Manganese	0.419 mg

CREAMY RED PEPPER SOUP

SERVES	PREP TIME	COOK TIME	READY IN
6	15 min	37 min	52 min

ALLERGENS: coconut   **Vegan**

NOTES: This soup has a warm but tangy flavor that makes the palate sing. These vegetables also provide an array of vitamins and nutrients that are perfect for boosting the immune system and giving your body some valuable phytonutrients.

INGREDIENTS

- 2 Tbsp olive oil
- 4 red bell peppers
- 1–16 oz bag of baby carrots, chopped
- 1 onion
- 3 cloves garlic
- 16 oz broth, unsalted
- 2 tsp salt
- 1/4 tsp pepper
- 1/2 cup coconut cream*

*I generally get coconut cream by refrigerating 1 can of coconut milk and removing the solidified cream at the top. Save remaining milk for another use.

DIRECTIONS

1. In a large pot heat the oil over medium-high heat. Place the onion and garlic in the pot and sauté for 2 minutes. Add the bell peppers and carrots and continue to sauté for an additional 5 minutes. Add the broth, salt, and pepper to the pot and bring to a boil. Reduce the heat to low, cover, and simmer for 30 minutes.
2. Transfer to a powerful blender and add the coconut cream. Puree until smooth. Add additional broth if you desire a thinner consistency. Garnish with coconut cream, nuts or seeds.

SWEET TREATS

Rich Cream & Berries, 189

Almond Butter Cups, 191

Chocolate Almond Butter Dip, 193

Almond Butter Caramels, 195

Best Grain-Free Chocolate Cake, 197

Peach Strawberry Crumble, 199

Rich Cream & Berries

NUTRITION INFORMATION

Serving Size: 1 Serving

Nutrient	Quantity	Nutrient	Quantity
Calories	449 kcal	Vitamin B-6	0.205 mg
Carbohydrates	26.88 g	Vitamin B-12 (Cobalamin)	0 µg
Fiber	3.3 g	Vitamin A	5 IU
Sugars	12.7 g	Vitamin E	0.89 mg
Starch	8.82 g	Vitamin D	0 IU
Total Fat	37.37 g	Vitamin K	13.6 µg
Omega 3	0.047 g	Calcium	27 mg
Omega 6	3.174 g	Magnesium	131 mg
Monounsaturated Fat	9.825 g	Phosphorus	305 mg
Protein	9.3 g	Iron	4.07 mg
Vitamin C	24.3 mg	Potassium	506 mg
Folate	33 µg	Sodium	8 mg
Vitamin B-1 (Thiamin)	0.186 mg	Zinc	2.82 mg
Vitamin B-2 (Riboflavin)	0.034 mg	Copper	1.072 mg
Vitamin B-3 (Niacin)	0.034 mg	Selenium	7.7 µg
Vitamin B-5 (Pantothenic acid)	1.092 mg	Manganese	1.558 mg

RICH CREAM & BERRIES

SERVES	PREP TIME	CHILL TIME	READY IN
4	20 min	4 hrs	4 hrs 20 min

ALLERGENS: cashew, coconut   **Vegan Adaptable**

NOTES: I typically find that the most simple dishes are the most gratifying. This rich and easy-to-make cream pairs perfectly with fresh fruit or homemade granola.

INGREDIENTS

- 1 cup cashews
- 1 cup coconut cream
- 2 Tbsp honey
- Fresh berries

DIRECTIONS

1. Place the cashews in a small saucepan and cover with water. Over high heat, boil the cashews for 15 minutes or until they crumble easily between your fingers when pressed.
2. Drain the water and place it in a powerful blender. Add the coconut cream and honey. Puree on high until the mixture is completely smooth.
3. Pour the cream into a medium glass bowl, cover, and refrigerate until chilled and thickened, about 4 hours.
4. Serve chilled with fresh berries.

Almond Butter Cups

NUTRITION INFORMATION

Serving Size: 1 Serving

Nutrient	Quantity	Nutrient	Quantity
Calories	590 kcal	Vitamin B-6	0.028 mg
Carbohydrates	45.37 g	Vitamin B-12 (Cobalamin)	0.02 µg
Fiber	4.4 g	Vitamin A	312 IU
Sugars	37.12 g	Vitamin E	0.34 mg
Starch	0 g	Vitamin D	7 IU
Total Fat	50.61 g	Vitamin K	1.4 µg
Omega 3	0.039 g	Calcium	22 mg
Omega 6	1.025 g	Magnesium	70 mg
Monounsaturated Fat	5.492 g	Phosphorus	109 mg
Protein	2.84 g	Iron	2.44 mg
Vitamin C	0.3 mg	Potassium	389 mg
Folate	6 µg	Sodium	183 mg
Vitamin B-1 (Thiamin)	0.017 mg	Zinc	1.02 mg
Vitamin B-2 (Riboflavin)	0.088 mg	Copper	0.534 mg
Vitamin B-3 (Niacin)	0.405 mg	Selenium	2.4 µg
Vitamin B-5 (Pantothenic acid)	0.081 mg	Manganese	0.574 mg

ALMOND BUTTER CUPS

SERVES	PREP TIME	COOK TIME	CHILL TIME
6	5 min	10 min	1 hr 10 min

ALLERGENS: almonds, coconut

NOTES: Be prepared for praise with these glorious little cups of all-natural goodness. They really are more delicious than their commercial comparable if you're asking me . . . and anyone else who's ever tried them.

INGREDIENTS

Chocolate:
- 1 cup coconut oil
- 1 cup cacao
- 2/3 cup honey

Filling:
- 1/3 cup almond butter
- 1 Tbsp coconut oil
- 2 Tbsp honey
- 1/2 Tbsp coconut flour
- 1/4 tsp salt

DIRECTIONS

1. Line a muffin tin with 12 paper liners.
2. Melt the coconut oil in a medium-size saucepan over medium heat. Once melted, remove from heat and whisk in the honey and cacao until thoroughly combined. Spoon 1 Tbsp of chocolate mixture into each liner. Set remaining chocolate aside. Place the muffin tin in the freezer for 10 minutes or until chocolate is hardened.
3. Meanwhile, combine all filling ingredients with an electric mixer until smooth. Remove frozen chocolate from the freezer. Spoon 1/2 Tbsp of filling mixture onto the center of each chocolate. Pour another 1 Tbsp of chocolate mixture over the filling. The filling should be completely covered. If any is emerging from the top press down slightly until chocolate covers it. Refrigerate until solid, about 1 hour.
4. Store the almond butter cups in an an airtight container in the refrigerator.

Chocolate Almond Butter Dip

NUTRITION INFORMATION

Serving Size: 1 Serving

Nutrient	Quantity	Nutrient	Quantity
Calories	334 kcal	Vitamin B-6	0.108 mg
Carbohydrates	28.76 g	Vitamin B-12 (Cobalamin)	0.08 µg
Fiber	2.1 g	Vitamin A	721 IU
Sugars	18.72 g	Vitamin E	0.7 mg
Starch	0 g	Vitamin D	17 IU
Total Fat	25.11 g	Vitamin K	2.6 µg
Omega 3	0.09 g	Calcium	70 mg
Omega 6	0.701 g	Magnesium	17 mg
Monounsaturated Fat	6.153 g	Phosphorus	58 mg
Protein	1.98 g	Iron	0.64 mg
Vitamin C	3.3 mg	Potassium	164 mg
Folate	10 µg	Sodium	342 mg
Vitamin B-1 (Thiamin)	0.068 mg	Zinc	0.66 mg
Vitamin B-2 (Riboflavin)	0.042 mg	Copper	0.091 mg
Vitamin B-3 (Niacin)	0.089 mg	Selenium	2.7 µg
Vitamin B-5 (Pantothenic acid)	0.175 mg	Manganese	0.197 mg

CHOCOLATE ALMOND BUTTER DIP

SERVES	PREP TIME	COOK TIME	READY IN
8	10 min	0 hrs	10 min

ALLERGENS: almonds, coconut   **Vegan Adaptable**

NOTES: Use this dip with some fresh fruit, homemade graham crackers, or cookies. You can also add a little extra almond or coconut milk and spread it over a cake. The flavor of this frosting is dark and rich. Feel free to add more honey if you prefer it a bit sweeter.

INGREDIENTS

- 1 cup almond butter
- 1 cup cacao powder
- 1/2 cup honey
- 1/4 cup coconut milk
- 1 Tbsp coconut oil
- 1/2 tsp salt

DIRECTIONS

1. Combine all ingredients with an electric hand mixer. The dip will be thick. You can add more milk if desired to get a thinner consistency.

Almond Butter Caramels

NUTRITION INFORMATION

Serving Size: 1 Serving

Nutrient	Quantity	Nutrient	Quantity
Calories	344 kcal	Vitamin B-6	0.008 mg
Carbohydrates	26.21 g	Vitamin B-12 (Cobalamin)	0.05 μg
Fiber	0.1 g	Vitamin A	709 IU
Sugars	26.12 g	Vitamin E	0.66 mg
Starch	0 g	Vitamin D	17 IU
Total Fat	28.11 g	Vitamin K	2 μg
Omega 3	0.088 g	Calcium	9 mg
Omega 6	0.705 g	Magnesium	1 mg
Monounsaturated Fat	6.261 g	Phosphorus	8 mg
Protein	0.34 g	Iron	0.14 mg
Vitamin C	0.2 mg	Potassium	23 mg
Folate	1 μg	Sodium	276 mg
Vitamin B-1 (Thiamin)	0.001 mg	Zinc	0.1 mg
Vitamin B-2 (Riboflavin)	0.022 mg	Copper	0.12 mg
Vitamin B-3 (Niacin)	0.05 mg	Selenium	0.5 μg
Vitamin B-5 (Pantothenic acid)	0.053 mg	Manganese	0.026 mg

ALMOND BUTTER CARAMELS

SERVES	PREP TIME	COOK TIME	CHILL TIME
8	5 min	15 min	15 min

ALLERGENS: almonds, coconut

NOTES: These caramels are so simple to make and sacrifice no flavor. They also store well thus are perfect for an on-hand treat and gift-giving.

INGREDIENTS

- 3/4 cup honey
- 3 Tbsp coconut oil
- 1 cup almond butter
- 1/4 tsp salt
- Flaked sea salt

DIRECTIONS

1. Line an 8 x 8 pan with parchment paper.
2. In a medium-sized pot over medium-high heat, bring the honey and oil to boil. Immediately reduce heat to low and simmer for 15 minutes, stirring occasionally.
3. Remove from heat and mix in the almond butter and 1/4 tsp of salt with an electric mixer. Pour the mixture into the prepared pan. Spread evenly and sprinkle with flaked sea salt.
4. Place in the refrigerator for 15 minutes or until caramels are set well enough to cut and hold their shape. Cut into small desired shapes and sizes.
5. Store in an airtight container at room temperature.

Best Grain-Free Chocolate Cake

NUTRITION INFORMATION

Serving Size: 1 Serving

Nutrient	Quantity	Nutrient	Quantity
Calories	380 kcal	Vitamin B-6	0.253 mg
Carbohydrates	54.06 g	Vitamin B-12 (Cobalamin)	0.95 µg
Fiber	4.1 g	Vitamin A	4713 IU
Sugars	37.85 g	Vitamin E	0.5 mg
Starch	0.4 g	Vitamin D	12 IU
Total Fat	18.47 g	Vitamin K	4.7 µg
Omega 3	0.319 g	Calcium	103 mg
Omega 6	1.815 g	Magnesium	36 mg
Monounsaturated Fat	2.271 g	Phosphorus	126 mg
Protein	5.22 g	Iron	1.82 mg
Vitamin C	6.6 mg	Potassium	376 mg
Folate	36 µg	Sodium	141 mg
Vitamin B-1 (Thiamin)	0.149 mg	Zinc	1.31 mg
Vitamin B-2 (Riboflavin)	0.128 mg	Copper	0.21 mg
Vitamin B-3 (Niacin)	0.463 mg	Selenium	9.8 µg
Vitamin B-5 (Pantothenic acid)	0.595 mg	Manganese	0.461 mg

BEST GRAIN-FREE CHOCOLATE CAKE

SERVES	PREP TIME	COOK TIME	COOL TIME
8	10 min	40 min	10 min

ALLERGENS: coconut, eggs, walnuts

NOTES: This really is the best whole food, grain-free chocolate cake ever. Make this a tiered cake, muffins, or a sheet cake. It really doesn't matter so long as it's smothered in ganache!

INGREDIENTS

- 2 cups raw carrots, chopped
- 2 eggs
- 1/2 cup coconut oil, melted
- 1/2 cup honey
- 1/4 cup coconut flour
- 3/4 cup cacao powder
- 1/4 tsp sea salt
- 1 tsp baking soda
- 2 tsp apple cider vinegar
- 1/3 cup walnuts, chopped

Ganache:
- 1 cup coconut cream
- 2/3 cup cacao powder
- 1/2 cup honey

DIRECTIONS

1. Preheat your oven to 350 °F. Grease 2–8" round pans liberally with coconut oil.
2. Place the carrots, eggs, oil, honey, flour, cacao, and salt into a powerful blender and puree until completely smooth.
3. Add baking soda and vinegar and blend until just barely incorporated. Fold in the walnuts.
4. Divide the batter evenly between two pans.
5. Bake for 20 minutes or until the tops are firm. Allow to cool for at least 10 minutes before turning out.
6. Meanwhile, combine all ganache ingredients in a medium saucepan over medium heat. Remove from heat once combined, creamy, and warmed through. Pour 1/4 cup of ganache on top of the first layer. Place the top layer of cake on and drizzle over the warm cake.

Peach Strawberry Crumble

NUTRITION INFORMATION

Serving Size: 1 Serving

Nutrient	Quantity	Nutrient	Quantity
Calories	109 kcal	Vitamin B-6	0.047 mg
Carbohydrates	7.33 g	Vitamin B-12 (Cobalamin)	0 µg
Fiber	1.3 g	Vitamin A	7 IU
Sugars	5.55 g	Vitamin E	0.18 mg
Starch	0.07 g	Vitamin D	0 IU
Total Fat	9.13 g	Vitamin K	0.8 µg
Omega 3	0.469 g	Calcium	12 mg
Omega 6	2.862 g	Magnesium	17 mg
Monounsaturated Fat	2.758 g	Phosphorus	36 mg
Protein	1.34 g	Iron	.37 mg
Vitamin C	14.2 mg	Potassium	79 mg
Folate	11 µg	Sodium	52 mg
Vitamin B-1 (Thiamin)	0.057 mg	Zinc	0.42 mg
Vitamin B-2 (Riboflavin)	0.02 mg	Copper	0.148 mg
Vitamin B-3 (Niacin)	0.208 mg	Selenium	0.5 µg
Vitamin B-5 (Pantothenic acid)	0.103 mg	Manganese	0.49 mg

PEACH STRAWBERRY CRUMBLE

SERVES	PREP TIME	COOK TIME	CHILL TIME
6	5 min	30 min	45 min

ALLERGENS: coconut, pecans, walnuts   **Vegan Adaptable**

NOTES: This is such an easy and delicious recipe, and a great way to use up any ripe summer peaches from your tree or local farmers' market.

INGREDIENTS

- 6 peaches, peeled and sliced
- 1 cup strawberries, tops removed and quartered
- 1/2 Tbsp honey
- 1/3 cup walnuts
- 1/3 cup pecans
- 2 Tbsp coconut sugar
- 1 Tbsp coconut oil, melted
- 1/8 tsp salt

DIRECTIONS

1. Preheat the oven to 350 °F.
2. Place the prepared peaches and strawberries in a 9 x 9 glass baking dish. Drizzle with the honey.
3. In a food processor, blend together the nuts, coconut sugar, coconut oil, and salt until fine and crumbly. Sprinkle over the fruit.
4. Place in the preheated oven for 30 minutes. Serve warm with lightly sweetened coconut cream or coconut ice cream.

Allowed and Non-Permitted Food List

A

Food	Permitted	Details
Acorn Squash	Yes	
Acacia	No	May be added in after a couple of months. Watch for symptoms
Agar-agar	No	Contains polysaccharides
Agave syrup	No	
Algae (Spirulina)	No	Can aggravate the immune system. May introduce later
Allspice	Yes	Spice only, not oil
Almond butter	Yes	Be sure there is no sugar or soybean oil
Almond milk	Yes	Introduce slowly, watch for tolerance. Check ingredients if store-bought
Almond oil	Yes	

Almonds	Yes	Eat sparingly to avoid constipation
Aloe vera	No	Contains polysaccharides and can cause GI inflammation and immune response
Amaranth	No	Grain and starch
Anchovies	Yes	
Apple cider	Yes	
Apple juice	Yes	100% juice. Look for "no sugar added" on the label
Apples	Yes	
Apricots	Yes	
Arrowroot	No	Starch
Artichoke (French)	Yes	Green exterior with partially edible leaves and edible heart
Artichoke (Jerusalem)	No	Starch. Brown and looks like a root
Ascorbic acid	Yes	
Asparagus	Yes	

Aspartame	No	Neurotoxin
Aspartic acid	No	Possible negative impact on liver, kidneys, and cholesterol
Avocado oil	Yes	
Avocados	Yes	

B

Food	Permitted	Details
Bananas	Yes	Be sure they are ripe with plenty of brown spots
Barley	No	
Bay leaf	Yes	
Bean flour	No	
Bean sprouts	No	
Beef	No	Difficult to digest. Also contains neurotoxic and inflammatory properties. Not a sustainable source
Beer	No	
Beets	Yes	
Berries	Yes	

Black Beans	No	Try during Phase Two. Slowly introduce when all digestive ailments have subsided. Soak overnight. Watch for tolerance
Blackeyed peas	No	
Bluefish	No	High mercury levels
Bok choy	Yes	
Bologna	No	
Bouillon cubes	No	Usually contains MSG or other harmful ingredients
Brandy	No	
Brazil nuts	Yes	Be sure they do not contain soybean oil or sugar
Broccoli	Yes	
Brussel sprouts	Yes	
Buckwheat	No	Grain
Bulgur	No	Grain
Butter	No	Casein

Butter beans	No	
Buttermilk	No	
Butternut squash	Yes	

C

Food	Permitted	Details
Cabbage	Yes	Slowly introduce when all digestive ailments have subsided. Watch for tolerance
Cacao	Yes	Ideally, introduce when most digestive ailments have subsided. Watch for digestive and behavioral tolerance
Calamari	Yes	
Cane juice	No	
Cannellini beans	No	
Cane sugar	No	
Canned fish	Yes	Only canned in water
Canned fruit	Yes	Only if canned in their own juice. No sugar or syrups

Canned vegetables	Yes	Fresh or frozen are preferable. Make sure only permitted ingredients are listed on the label
Canola oil	Yes	Not ideal
Cantaloupe	Yes	
Capers	Yes	
Carob	Yes	
Carrageenan	No	High in polysaccharides
Carrots	Yes	
Cashews	Yes	Be sure they do not contain soybean oil or sugar
Casein	No	Inflammatory and neurotoxic properties
Cauliflower	Yes	Slowly introduce when most digestive ailments have subsided. Watch for tolerance

Celery root	Yes	Highly fibrous. Slowly introduce when most digestive ailments have subsided. Watch for tolerance
Celery	Yes	
Cellulose	Yes	
Cellulose gum	No	
Cereal	No	
Chard	Yes	
Cheese	No	Casein
Cherries	Yes	
Chestnuts	Yes	Slowly introduce when most digestive ailments have subsided. Watch for tolerance
Chewing gum	No	
Chia seeds	No	Has mucilaginous gel and is not conducive to GI healing
Chicken	Yes	

Chickpeas	No	Can try in Phase Two. Slowly introduce when all digestive ailments have subsided. Soak overnight. Watch for tolerance
Chicory root	No	Contains saccharides
Cilantro	Yes	
Cinnamon	Yes	
Citric acid	Yes	
Club soda	Yes	
Cocoa powder	No	Look for pure cacao instead
Coconut	Yes	
Coconut milk	Yes	Be sure there are no non-approved added ingredients
Coconut oil	Yes	
Coconut sugar	Yes	Watch for tolerance
Cod	Yes	Sparingly. Can contain moderate mercury

Coffee	Yes	Fresh, not instant
Collard greens	Yes	Slowly introduce when most digestive ailments have subsided. Watch for digestive tolerance
Corn	No	Anything with corn is not permitted. This includes the vegetable, popcorn, and corn flour
Corn oil	Yes	Not ideal
Corn syrup	No	
Corn starch	No	
Cottage cheese	No	
Couscous	No	Grain
Crab	Yes	
Cranberry juice	Yes	Look for "no sugar added". May be sweetened with apple juice or honey
Cream	No	
Cream cheese	No	

Foods Four Thought Diet

Cream of tartar	No	
Croaker fish	No	High mercury levels
Cucumbers	Yes	

D

Food	Permitted	Details
Date sugar	Yes	Watch for tolerance
Dates	Yes	No added ingredients
Decaf products	No	
Dextrose	No	
Dried milk	No	
Durum flour	No	

E

Food	Permitted	Details
Echinacea	Yes	Good for immunity
Eggplant	Yes	
Eggs	Yes	This is a common allergy food. Keep it on your radar. If a suspected allergy exists, eliminate these. Watch for symptoms
Ezekiel bread	No	Sprouted grain

F

Food	Permitted	Details
Fava beans	No	
Farro	No	Grain seed
Fenugreek	No	
Figs	Yes	Highly laxative. Slowly introduce when most digestive ailments have subsided. Watch for tolerance
Fish	Yes	Mostly okay. Ideally fresh or frozen. Be sure nothing has been added
Flaxseed	No	Often causes diarrhea or other problems with the stool. May be slowly introduced after digestive ailments have subsided
Flaxseed oil	Yes	
Flour	No	

Freekeh	No	Grain
Frozen orange juice (concentrated)	No	Any juice from concentrate should not be consumed. Often contains sugars not listed
Fructose	No	
Fruit (canned)	Yes	Only if canned in 100% own juice, no sugar or concentrate

G

Food	Permitted	Details
Garbanzo beans	No	Try in Phase Two. Slowly introduce when all digestive ailments have subsided. Soak overnight. Watch for tolerance
Garlic	Yes	
Gelatin (unflavored)	Yes	
Ghee	Yes	
Ginger	Yes	
Glucose	No	
Glycerin	Yes	
Grape juice	Yes	100% juice. Look for label to say "no sugar added"
Grapefruit	Yes	
Grapefruit juice	Yes	Typically only fresh. Most store-bought contains sugar
Grapes	Yes	

Grapeseed oil	Yes	
Green tea	Yes	
Grouper fish	No	High mercury levels
Guar gum	No	Product of corn, thus a starch
Gums	No	

H

Food	Permitted	Details
Halibut	No	Moderate to high levels of mercury
Ham	No	Pork is typically more difficult to digest. May be introduced slowly when GI symptoms have passed. Watch for tolerance. Not a sustainable food source
Haricot beans	No	May try in Phase Two. Slowly introduce when all digestive ailments have subsided. Soak overnight. Watch for tolerance
Hazelnuts	Yes	
Hemp seed, hemp protein	No	
Honey	Yes	

Horseradish sauce	No	Can be harsh on the intestine. Often contains non-approved ingredients
Hot dogs	No	I have only ever found one approved hot dog brand in the grocery store. Most have harmful fillers, flavors, or sugar
Hydrolyzed protein	No	Neurotoxic properties

I

Food	Permitted	Details
Ice cream	No	Commercially prepared always has non-approved items. You may however make your own with approved ingredients
Inositol	No	Sugar alcohol
Inulin	No	Sugar substance
Isoglucose	No	Sugar substance

J

Food	Permitted	Details
Jalapenos	Yes	Consider introducing when GI symptoms have subsided. Watch for tolerance
Jicama	No	Starchy root
Juice from concentrate	No	Concentrated food items often have added ingredients that are not required to be listed, most often sugar

K

Food	Permitted	Details
Kale	Yes	
Kefir	No	
Ketchup	No	Typically contains sugar. Tomatoes are also a natural neurotoxic food so should be consumed sparingly
Kidney beans	No	May be introduced in Phaase Two
Kimchi	Yes	
Kiwi	Yes	
Kohlrabi	No	May be introduced when GI symptoms have subsided. Watch for tolerance
Kudzu	No	Starch
Kumquats	Yes	

L

Food	Permitted	Details
L-theanine	Yes	Check the label for non-approved fillers
Lamb	Yes	
Lecithin	No	Typically seen listed as soy lecithin
Leek	Yes	
Lemons	Yes	
Lentils	No	Try in Phase two. Slowly introduce when all digestive ailments have subsided. Soak overnight. Watch for tolerance
Lettuce	Yes	
Leucine	Yes	
Licorice	No	Laxative effect

Lima beans	No	Try in Phase Two. Slowly introduce when all digestive ailments have subsided. Soak overnight. Watch for tolerance
Limes	Yes	
Liqueurs	No	
Lobster	Yes	Sparingly. Contains moderate mercury

M

Food	Permitted	Details
Macadamia nuts	Yes	
Macadamia oil	Yes	
Mackerel	No	Moderate to high mercury levels
Magnesium citrate	Yes	
Magnesium stearate	Yes	
Mahi mahi	Yes	Sparingly. Contains moderate mercury
Maltitol	No	Sugar alcohol
Maltodextrin	No	Derived from starch
Mangoes	Yes	
Mannitol	No	Sugar alcohol
Maple syrup	No	Disaccharide
Margarine	No	
Marlin	No	High mercury levels

Marshmallow root	No	Mucilaginous herb. Can irritate digestive symptoms. May be added in later. Watch for GI symptoms
Mastic gum	No	
Mead	No	
Melon	Yes	
Milk	No	
Millet	No	Grain seed
Miso	No	
Molasses	No	
Monkfish	Yes	Sparingly. Contains moderate mercury
MSG	No	Extreme neurotoxin
Mung beans	No	
Mushrooms	No	Natural Neurotoxin. Eat sparingly after Phase One.
Mustard	Yes	Typically approved. Check ingredients carefully

N

Food	Permitted	Details
Natural flavors	No	Can refer to anything and does not mean chemical-free
Navy beans	No	Try in Phase Two. Slowly introduce when all digestive ailments have subsided. Soak overnight. Watch for tolerance
Nectarines	Yes	
Nettle	Yes	Watch for side effects
Nutmeg	Yes	

O

Food	Permitted	Details
Oats	No	
Okra	No	Mucilaginous food
Olive oil	Yes	
Olives	Yes	Make sure the ingredients list is approved items
Onions	Yes	Avoid onion powder. This typically has anti-caking ingredients that are non-approved
Orange juice	Yes	Be sure there is no sugar added
Orange roughy	No	High mercury levels
Oranges	Yes	
Oregano	Yes	
Oyster	Yes	

P

Food	Permitted	Details
Papayas	Yes	
Paprika	Yes	
Parsley	Yes	
Parsnips	No	Sometimes not tolerated well. Try adding them in once GI symptoms have subsided
Passion fruit	Yes	
Pasta	No	
Pea flour	No	
Peaches	Yes	
Peanut butter	No	An inflammatory food. You may try after several months of strict dieting. Check ingredients closely. Many contain sugar and soybean oil
Peanut oil	No	Same rules as peanut butter

Peanuts	No	Same rules as peanut butter
Pears	Yes	
Peas	No	Natural neurotoxic properties. Also a starch. Eliminate entirely during the diet. You may introduce and eat sparingly forever after
Pecans	Yes	
Pectin	No	Occurs naturally in many fruits, however, in concentrated doses, the body responds to it as it would a complex sugar
Peppermint	Yes	
Peppers	Yes	
Perch fish	No	High mercury levels
Persimmons	Yes	
Pickles	Yes	Dill is allowed
Pine nuts	Yes	

Pineapple	Yes	
Pineapple juice	Yes	Check for added ingredients
Pinto beans	No	
Pistachio nuts	Yes	Check ingredients closely. Some contain starch, dyes, or soybean oil
Plantains	No	Too starchy
Plums	Yes	
Polysorbate	No	
Pomegranate	Yes	
Poppyseed	Yes	
Pork	No	Typically more difficult on digestion compared to other forms of meat.
Port wine	No	
Postum	No	
Potassium sorbate	Yes	
Potatoes	No	

Poultry	Yes	Try to buy free-range. Check labels for ingredients
Prunes	Yes	
Psyllium husks	No	
Pumpkin	Yes	Check ingredients if canned

Q

Food	Permitted	Details
Quinoa	No	Grain seed and starch. May be introduced during Phase Two.
Quorn	No	

R

Food	Permitted	Details
Raisins	Yes	Check ingredients
Rhubarb	Yes	
Rice	No	Grain. This includes brown and white
Rice bran	No	
Rice flour	No	
Rosemary	Yes	
Rutabaga	Yes	
Rye	No	Grain

S

Food	Permitted	Details
Sablefish	No	High mercury levels
Saccharine	Yes	
Safflower oil	Yes	Not ideal
Sage	Yes	
Sago starch	No	
Sake	No	
Salmon	Yes	This is the best fish option. Buy wild Alaskan
Sardines	Yes	
Scallop	Yes	
Sea bass	No	High mercury levels
Sesame seeds	Yes	
Shark	No	High mercury levels
Shrimp	Yes	
Snapper	Yes	Sparingly. Contains moderate mercury
Sole	Yes	

Sorghum	No	Grain
Stevia	No	Can cause discomfort in some. Add in once healing is obtained
Swordfish	No	High mercury levels

T

Food	Permitted	Details
Tabasco sauce	Yes	Check the labels for added sugar or gums
Tahini	Yes	
Tamarii	No	Soy
Tamarind	No	Legume
Tangerines	Yes	
Tapioca	No	Starch
Taro	No	Too much starch
Tarragon	Yes	
Tea	Yes	Use caution. Check labels
Teff	No	Grain seed
Thyme	Yes	
Tilapia	No	This fish is usually farmed and low in quality
Tofu	No	Soy
Tofutti cheese	No	

Tomato	No	Natural Neurotoxin. Eat sparingly after Phase One.
Triticale	No	Grain
Trout	Yes	
Tuna	No	Moderate to high levels of mercury
Turbinado	No	Cane sugar
Turnip	No	Sometimes not tolerated well. Try adding them in once GI symptoms have subsided

V

Food	Permitted	Details
V8	No	
Vanilla	No	The bean in pure form is entirely acceptable. However, most vanilla extract contains sugar, alcohol, gums, and colors. There are few pure bottled forms and they are quite expensive
Vegetable stearate	Yes	
Vegetables (canned)	Yes	Fresh or frozen are preferable
Vinegar	Yes	Apple cider vinegar is particularly excellent

W

Food	Permitted	Details
Walnut oil	Yes	
Walnuts	Yes	Check ingredients. Should not contain added oils
Wasabi	Yes	Check ingredients for fillers
Water chestnuts	No	
Watercress	Yes	
Watermelon	Yes	
Wheat	No	Grain
Wheat berry	No	Grain
Wheat germ	No	
Wine	No	

X

Food	Permitted	Details
Xanthan gum	No	
Xylitol	No	Sugar alcohol

Y

Food	Permitted	Details
Yams	No	
Yogurt	No	
Yogurt (homemade)	No	Still can contain casein. However, a potentially good to reintroduce later on
Yucca root	No	

Z

Food	Permitted	Details
Zucchini	Yes	

Additional Resources

Websites for Healthy Lifestyle

Mind Body Green
www.mindbodygreen.com

Clean Eating Magazine
www.cleaneatingmag.com

Mark's Daily Apple
www.marksdailyapple.com

Mommypotamus
www.mommypotamus.com

Wellness Mama
www.wellnessmama.com

Dr. Axe
www.draxe.com

Meditation Tools

Mindful
www.mindful.org

Headspace
www.headspace.com

Tiny Buddha
www.tinybuddha.com

Mindfulness Coach App

Compliant or Easily Modified Recipes

Foods Four Thought
www.foodsfourthought.com

Against All Grain
www.againstallgrain.com

AIP Paleo
www.autoimmunewellness.com

Detoxinista
www.detoxinista.com

The Paleo Mom
www.thepaleomom.com

FFT Approved Products

Almonds and Almond Butter: Wild Soil Almonds
www.wildsoilalmonds.com

Almond Flour: Bob's Red Mill
www.bobsredmill.com

Apple Cider Vinegar: Bragg
www.bragg.com

Cacao Powder: Healthworks
www.healthworks.com

Coconut Aminos: Coconut Secret
www.coconutsecret.com

Coconut Flour, Sugar, and Oil: Nutiva
www.nutiva.com

Coconut Milk: Golden Star
Find their products on Walmart.com or Amazon.com

Collagen and Gelatin: Great Lakes Gelatin
www.greatlakesgelatin.com

Deli Meat: Applegate
www.applegate.com

Ghee: Organic Valley
www.organicvalley.coop

Honey: Nature Nate
www.naturenates.com

Nut Milk: Elmhurst
www.elmhurst1925.com

Tahini: Baron's
Find their products on Walmart.com or Amazon.com

Freeze Dried Fruit: Crispy Green (On-the-Go)
www.crispygreen.com

Freeze Dried Fruit: Homegrown Organic Farms (On-the-Go)
Find their products on Amazon.com

Fruit & Vegetable Squeezers: Happy Family Organics (On the-Go)
www.happyfamilyorganics.com

Fruit & Vegetable Squeezers: GoGo Squeez (On-the-Go)
www.gogosqueez.com

Nut Mix: Daily Fresh (On-the-Go)
Find their products on Walmart.com or Amazon.com

Snack Bars: LaraBar (On-the-Go)
www.larabar.com

Snack Bars and Nut Butter: RXBar (On-the-Go)
www.rxbar.com

Supplement Sources

Fish Oil: Fermented Cod Liver Oil
www.greenpasture.org

Fish Oil: DHA BrainCare
www.vitalchoice.com

Magnesium Glycinate
www.pureencapsulations.com

Multi-Vitamin
www.newchapter.com

Zinc Chelate
www.puremicronutrients.com

Probiotic: Latero-Flora
www.globalhealing.com

Probiotic: Complete Probiotics Platinum
www.1md.org

Other Good Supplements
www.holisticheal.com
www.bodyecology.com

Organization

KonMari
www.konmari.com

I Heart Organizing
www.iheartorganizing.com

Good Housekeeping
www.goodhousekeeping.com

Additional Learning

Additude: Inside the ADHD Mind
www.additudemag.com

American Autoimmune Related Diseases Association
www.aarda.org

Autism Support Network
www.autismsupportnetwork.com

Sharing Your Success Story

I love hearing about your family's victories and stories of growth. It's truly such a gift. There are several ways you can share your Foods Four Thought story, and I promise if you send it in privately I'll secure your express permission before sharing any part of it.

Email
crystal@foodsfourthought.com
Send me your story, along with your name, city, state, and any photography if you'd like. I will turn these emails into features on the Foods Four Thought testimonial page.

Instagram
@foodsfourthought and #foodsfourthought
Show us your victories, either little or big, while on the FFT journey. I'd love to feature you on the feed.

Facebook
Share your story or photos on the Foods Four Thought Facebook wall, or tag @foodsfourthought

Book Review
Share your review of the book and the program wherever you purchased it. This will help other parents like yourself find

confidence as they consider endeavoring in the journey, and of course, this helps me as the author, XO.

References

1. Adams, James B et al. "Gastrointestinal flora and gastrointestinal status in children with autism--comparisons to typical children and correlation with autism severity." BMC gastroenterology vol. 11 22. 16 Mar. 2011, doi:10.1186/1471-230X-11-22.

2. Albertson, E.R., Neff, K.D. & Dill-Shackleford, K.E. Self-Compassion and Body Dissatisfaction in Women: A Randomized Controlled Trial of a Brief Meditation Intervention. Mindfulness 6, 444–454 (2015). https://doi.org/10.1007/s12671-014-0277-3.

3. Amminger, G. P., Berger, G. E., Schäfer, M. R., Klier, C., Friedrich, M. H., & Feucht, M. (2007). Omega-3 Fatty Acids Supplementation in Children with Autism: A Double-blind Randomized, Placebo-controlled Pilot Study. Biological Psychiatry, 61(4), 551–553.

4. Ardhanareeswaran, Karthikeyan, and Fred Volkmarb. "Autism Spectrum Disorders." Www.Ncbi.Nlm.Nih.Gov, Yale Journal of Biology and Medicine, 4 Mar. 2015, www.ncbi.nlm.nih.gov/pmc/articles/PMC4345536.

5. Ashwood, Paul, et al. "Intestinal Lymphocyte Populations in Children with Regressive Autism: Evidence for Extensive Mucosal Immunopathology." Journal of Clinical Immunology, vol. 23, no. 6, 2003, pp. 504–17. Crossref, doi:10.1023/b:joci.0000010427.05143.bb.

6. Atladottir, H. O., et al. "Association of Family History of Autoimmune Diseases and Autism Spectrum Disorders." PEDIATRICS, vol. 124, no. 2, 2009, pp. 687–94. Crossref, doi:10.1542/peds.2008-2445.

7. Bonaz, Bruno, et al. "The Vagus Nerve at the Interface of the Microbiota-Gut-Brain Axis." Frontiers in Neuroscience, vol. 12, 2018. Crossref, doi:10.3389/fnins.2018.00049.

8. Bonnie Raingruber & Carol Robinson (2007) The Effectiveness of Tai Chi, Yoga, Meditation, and Reiki Healing Sessions in Promoting Health and Enhancing Problem Solving Abilities of Registered Nurses, Issues in Mental Health Nursing, 28:10, 1141-1155, DOI: 10.1080/01612840701581255.

9. Bradbury J. (2011). Docosahexaenoic acid (DHA): an ancient nutrient for the modern human brain. Nutrients, 3(5), 529–554. https://doi.org/10.3390/nu3050529.

10. Brian Rees, MC USAR, Overview of Outcome Data of Potential Meditation Training for Soldier Resilience, Military Medicine, Volume 176, Issue 11, November 2011, Pages 1232–1242, https://doi.org/10.7205/MILMED-D-11-00067.

11. Ceccarelli, F., Agmon-Levin, N., & Perricone, C. (2017). Genetic Factors of Autoimmune Diseases 2017. Journal of immunology research, 2017, 2789242. https://doi.org/10.1155/2017/2789242.

12. "CDC Releases First Estimates of the Number of Adults Living with ASD." Centers for Disease Control and Prevention, 27 Apr. 2020, www.cdc.gov/ncbddd/autism/features/adults-living-with-autism-spectrum-disorder.html.

13. Chaidez, V., Hansen, R.L. & Hertz-Picciotto, I. Gastrointestinal Problems in Children with Autism, Developmental Delays or Typical Development. J Autism Dev Disord 44, 1117–1127 (2014). https: doi.org/10.1007/s10803-013-1973-x.

14. Chaidez, Virginia, et al. "Gastrointestinal Problems in Children with Autism, Developmental Delays or Typical Development." Journal of Autism and Developmental Disorders, vol. 44, no. 5, 2013, pp. 1117–27. Crossref, doi:10.1007/s10803-013-1973-x.

15. Chu, L.-C. (2010). The benefits of meditation vis-à-vis emotional intelligence, perceived stress and negative mental health. Stress and Health, 26(2), 169–180. https://doi.org/10.1002/smi.1289.

16. Clonan, A., Roberts, K., & Holdsworth, M. (2016). Socioeconomic and demographic drivers of red and processed meat consumption: Implications for health and environmental sustainability. *Proceedings of the Nutrition Society, 75*(3), 367-373. doi:10.1017/S0029665116000100

17. Coker TR, Chan LS, Newberry SJ, Limbos MA, Suttorp MJ, Shekelle PG, Takata GS. Diagnosis, microbial epidemiology, and antibiotic treatment of acute otitis media in children: a

systematic review. JAMA. 2010 Nov 17;304(19):2161-9. doi: 10.1001/jama.2010.1651. PMID: 21081729.

18. Comi AM, Zimmerman AW, Frye VH, Law PA, Peeden JN. Familial Clustering of Autoimmune Disorders and Evaluation of Medical Risk Factors in Autism. Journal of Child Neurology. 1999;14(6):388-394. doi:10.1177/088307389901400608.

19. "Data and Statistics on Autism Spectrum Disorder | CDC." Centers for Disease Control and Prevention, 25 Sept. 2020, www.cdc.gov/ncbddd/autism/data.html.

20. De Filippo, C., Cavalieri, D., Di Paola, M., Ramazzotti, M., Poullet, J. B., Massart, S., Collini, S., Pieraccini, G., & Lionetti, P. (2010). Impact of diet in shaping gut microbiota revealed by a comparative study in children from Europe and rural Africa. Proceedings of the National Academy of Sciences, 107(33), 14691–14696. https://doi.org/10.1073/pnas.1005963107.

21. Deepika Bagga, Johanna Louise Reichert, Karl Koschutnig, Christoph Stefan Aigner, Peter Holzer, Kaisa Koskinen, Christine Moissl-Eichinger & Veronika Schöpf (2018) Probiotics drive gut microbiome triggering emotional brain signatures, Gut Microbes, 9:6, 486-496, DOI: 10.1080/19490976.2018.1460015.

22. de Lemos ML. Effects of Soy Phytoestrogens Genistein and Daidzein on Breast Cancer Growth. Annals of Pharmacotherapy. 2001;35(9):1118-1121. doi:10.1345/aph.10257.

23. Dinan, T., Cryan, J. Brain–gut–microbiota axis — mood, metabolism and behaviour. Nat Rev Gastroenterol Hepatol 14, 69–70 (2017). https://doi.org/10.1038/nrgastro.2016.200.

24. Frye, R. E., et al. "Thyroid Dysfunction in Children with Autism Spectrum Disorder Is Associated with Folate Receptor α Autoimmune Disorder." Journal of Neuroendocrinology, vol. 29, no. 3, 2017. Crossref, doi:10.1111/jne.12461.

25. Gottschall, Elaine. "Digestion-Gut-Autism Connection: The Specific Carbohydrate Diet." Medical Veritas: The Journal of Medical Truth, vol. 1, 2004, pp. 261–71. Crossref, doi:10.1588/medver.2004.01.00029.

26. Harvard Health Publishing. "Can Gut Bacteria Improve Your Health?" Harvard Health, www.health.harvard.edu/staying-healthy/can-gut-bacteria-improve-your-health. Accessed 11 Oct. 2020.

27. Horvath, Karoly, et al. "Gastrointestinal Abnormalities in Children with Autistic Disorder." The Journal of Pediatrics, vol. 135, no. 5, 1999, pp. 559–63. Crossref, doi:10.1016/s0022-3476(99)70052-1.

28. Hsiao, Elaine Y., et al. "Microbiota Modulate Behavioral and Physiological Abnormalities Associated with Neurodevelopmental Disorders." Cell, vol. 155, no. 7, 2013, pp. 1451–63. Crossref, doi:10.1016/j.cell.2013.11.024.

29. Hsiao, E. Y., McBride, S. W., Hsien, S., Sharon, G., Hyde, E. R., McCue, T., Codelli, J. A., Chow, J., Reisman, S. E., Petrosino, J. F., Patterson, P. H., & Mazmanian, S. K. (2013). Microbiota Modulate Behavioral and Physiological Abnormalities Associated with Neurodevelopmental Disorders. Cell, 155(7), 1451–1463. https://doi.org/10.1016/j.cell.2013.11.024.

30. Hughes, H. K., Mills Ko, E., Rose, D., & Ashwood, P. (2018). Immune Dysfunction and Autoimmunity as Pathological Mechanisms in Autism Spectrum Disorders. Frontiers in cellular neuroscience, 12, 405. https://doi.org/10.3389/fncel.2018.00405.

31. Iossifov, Ivan, et al. "De Novo Gene Disruptions in Children on the Autistic Spectrum." Neuron, vol. 74, no. 2, 2012, pp. 285–99. Crossref, doi:10.1016/j.neuron.2012.04.009.

32. Kaul, Gastrointestinal Microflora Studies in Late-Onset Autism, Clinical Infectious Diseases, Volume 35, Issue Supplement_1, September 2002, Pages S6–S16, https://doi.org/10.1086/341914.

33. Klukowski M, Wasilewska J, Lebensztejn D. Sleep and gastrointestinal disturbances in autism spectrum disorder in children. Developmental Period Medicine. 2015 Apr-Jun;19(2):157-161.

34. Liang, Shan. "Gut-Brain Psychology: Rethinking Psychology From the Microbiota–Gut–Brain Axis." Frontiers, 11 Oct. 2020, www.frontiersin.org/articles/

10.3389/fnint.2018.00033/full.

35. Maenner MJ, Shaw KA, Baio J, et al. Prevalence of Autism Spectrum Disorder Among Children Aged 8 Years — Autism and Developmental Disabilities Monitoring Network, 11 Sites, United States, 2016. MMWR Surveill Summ 2020;69(No. SS-4):1–12. DOI: http://dx.doi.org/10.15585/mmwr.ss6904a1.

36. Matelski, Lauren, and Judy Van de Water. "Risk Factors in Autism: Thinking Outside the Brain." Journal of Autoimmunity, vol. 67, 2016, pp. 1–7. Crossref, doi:10.1016/j.jaut.2015.11.003.

37. Messaoudi, Michaël, et al. "Assessment of Psychotropic-like Properties of a Probiotic Formulation (Lactobacillus HelveticusR0052 AndBifidobacterium LongumR0175) in Rats and Human Subjects." British Journal of Nutrition, vol. 105, no. 5, 2010, pp. 755–64. Crossref, doi:10.1017/s0007114510004319.

38. Navarro, F., Pearson, D. A., Fatheree, N., Mansour, R., Hashmi, S. S., & Rhoads, J. M. (2014). Are 'leaky gut' and behavior associated with gluten and dairy containing diet in children with autism spectrum disorders? *Nutritional Neuroscience*, *18(4)*, 177-185. doi:10.1179/1476830514y.0000000110

39. Neuroscience News. "Gut Bacteria Influence Autism-like Behaviors in Mice." Neuroscience News, 30 May 2019, neurosciencenews.com/microbiome-behavior-asd-14124/#:%7E:text=New%20research%20shows%20that%20gut,meta

bolites%20or%20a%20probiotic%20drug.

40. Parmar, Nirav B., et al. "Composition of Ghee Prepared from Camel, Cow and Buffalo Milk." Journal of Camel Practice and Research, vol. 25, no. 3, 2018, p. 321. Crossref, doi:10.5958/2277-8934.2018.00046.2.

41. Phillips, Barry. "Otitis Media, Milk Allergy, and Folk Medicine." American Academy of Pediatrics, 1 Aug. 1972, pediatrics.aappublications.org/content/50/2/346.1.

42. "Probiotic Therapy Alleviates Autism-like Behaviors in Mice." California Institute of Technology, www.caltech.edu/about/news/probiotic-therapy-alleviates-autism-behaviors-mice-41306. Accessed 11 Oct. 2020.

43. Richard E. Frye, Shannon Rose, John Slattery & Derrick F. MacFabe (2015) Gastrointestinal dysfunction in autism spectrum disorder: the role of the mitochondria and the enteric microbiome, Microbial Ecology in Health and Disease, 26:1, DOI: 10.3402/mehd.v26.27458.

44. Sanaa Y. Shaaban, Yasmin G. El Gendy, Nayra S. Mehanna, Waled M. El-Senousy, Howaida S. A. El-Feki, Khaled Saad & Osama M. El-Asheer (2018) The role of probiotics in children with autism spectrum disorder: A prospective, open-label study, Nutritional Neuroscience, 21:9, 676-681, DOI: 10.1080/1028415X.2017.1347746.

45. Stettler, Nicolas, et al. "Systematic Review of Clinical Studies Related to Pork Intake and Metabolic Syndrome or Its Components." *Diabetes, Metabolic Syndrome and*

Obesity : Targets and Therapy, Dove Medical Press, 25 Sept. 2013, www.ncbi.nlm.nih.gov/pmc/articles/PMC3792009/.

46. Suskind, David L.; Wahbeh, Ghassan; Gregory, Nila; Vendettuoli, Heather; Christie, Dennis Nutritional Therapy in Pediatric Crohn Disease: The Specific Carbohydrate Diet, Journal of Pediatric Gastroenterology and Nutrition: January 2014 - Volume 58 - Issue 1 - p 87-91 doi: 10.1097/MPG.0000000000000103.

47. Sydney M. Finegold, Denise Molitoris, Yuli Song, Chengxu Liu, Marja-Liisa Vaisanen, Ellen Bolte, Maureen McTeague, Richard Sandler, Hannah Wexler, Elizabeth M. Marlowe, Matthew D. Collins, Paul A. Lawson, Paula Summanen, Mehmet Baysallar, Thomas J. Tomzynski, Erik Read, Eric Johnson, Rial Rolfe, Palwasha Nasir, Haroun Shah, David A. Haake, Patricia Manning, Ajay.

48. Tayama, J., Ogawa, S., Nakaya, N., Sone, T., Hamaguchi, T., Takeoka, A., Hamazaki, K., Okamura, H., Yajima, J., Kobayashi, M., Hayashida, M., & Shirabe, S. (2019). Omega-3 polyunsaturated fatty acids and psychological intervention for workers with mild to moderate depression: A double-blind randomized controlled trial. Journal of Affective Disorders, 245, 364–370. https://doi.org/10.1016/j.jad.2018.11.039.

49. "The Association of Environmental Toxicants and Autism Spectrum Disorders in Children." ScienceDirect, 1 Aug. 2017, www.sciencedirect.com/science/article/abs/pii/S0269749116327713.

50. Vojdani, Aristo. "A Potential Link between Environmental Triggers and Autoimmunity." Autoimmune Diseases, vol. 2014, 2014, pp. 1–18. Crossref, doi:10.1155/2014/437231.

51. Wang, L., Yu, Y., Zhang, Y. et al. Hydrogen breath test to detect small intestinal bacterial overgrowth: a prevalence case–control study in autism. Eur Child Adolesc Psychiatry 27, 233–240 (2018). https://doi.org/10.1007/s00787-017-1039-2.

52. Zhu, S., Jiang, Y., Xu, K. et al. The progress of gut microbiome research related to brain disorders. J Neuroinflammation 17, 25 (2020). https://doi.org/10.1186/s12974-020-1705-z.

Index

A

Absorption 38-39

ADHD 1, 7, 16, 20, 26-28

Alcohol 40

Allergies 28, 31, 40-41, 93

Animal Protein 44, 47-49, 85

Antibiotics 23-24

Anxiety 20-21, 54

Autism (ASD) 1, 5, 7, 13-14, 16, 20-21, 23, 26-28

Autoimmune Disorder 1, 7, 16-17, 19-20, 28

B

Bacteria 20-25, 27, 31-32, 40, 44, 52-53, 76

Banana 45-46, 105, 112

Barley 38, 87, 196

Beans 32, 34, 38, 42, 51, 85, 87

Behavior 2-3, 7, 14-15, 20-24, 26, 30-35, 38, 77, 80, 85, 87

Buckwheat 38, 87, 197

C

Cabbage 44, 199

Calories 46, 74, 76

Candida 21, 23, 32

Carbohydrate 15, 25-27, 31-32, 41, 76

Casein 14, 26-27, 41, 87

Cheese 41, 87, 201

Colonic Disease 25

Constipation 20, 47

Corn 32, 38, 44, 48, 87, 203

Crohn's disease 27-28

Cruciferous 45

D

Dairy 41-42, 85

Detoxification 83

Diarrhea 15, 20, 25, 44-45, 53

Digestion 33, 38, 44-45, 48

Disaccharides 25

E

Eggs 32, 47-48, 69, 77

Enzyme 31

F

Fatigue 20

Fats 29, 42, 46, 74

Ferment 44, 53

Fiber 25, 37, 43

Flour 46, 106-107

Fruit 29, 32, 28, 42, 44-46, 77, 85, 105

G

Gases 22, 47, 52, 83

Genetics 19

Glutamate 42

Gluten 15, 26-27, 34, 48, 51, 87

Grains 27, 32, 34, 38, 55, 78

Gut 3, 21-22, 24-26, 31, 52, 74

H

Herbs 45

Honey 33, 44, 49, 69, 211

Hyperactivity 1, 54

I

Immune system 3, 21, 41

Infection 21, 24, 31, 41

Inflammation 25-28, 30, 38, 40-41, 48

Intestinal flora 22, 25, 52

Intestinal mucosa 23

Intolerance 33, 42

L

Lactose 43

Leaky Gut 21, 24, 26

Lectins 42

Legumes 40-41, 53

Lentils 38, 87, 216

M

Malabsorption 21, 48

Malnutrition 23-24

Milk 24, 41, 87, 106-107

Mucus 25, 42

Mushrooms 42, 87, 219

N

Neurological 5, 20-22, 26, 43

Nuts 32, 38, 44, 46-47

O

Oats 38, 51, 87, 221

P

Parsnip 44, 222

Peanuts 38, 40, 223

Peas 38, 44, 87, 223

Potatoes 32, 44, 87, 224

Proteins 27, 29, 40-42, 44, 47-49, 51, 85

Psoriasis 28

Q

Quinoa 36, 40, 90, 92-93, 234

R

Rice 40, 54, 93, 235

Rye 40, 93, 235

S

Small intestine 20, 25

Soy 38-39, 47-48, 54, 66, 70, 87, 106

Specific carbohydrates 15-16, 26

Starch 26-27, 32, 44, 46

Stevia 49, 87, 229

Sugar 25-27, 32-33, 40, 44, 49, 66, 87, 106

Sweeteners, artificial 40, 52

T

Tofu 39, 87, 230

Tomatoes 42, 87

Toxic 21, 23, 25, 48

U

Underweight 46

V

Vagus nerve 24, 74

Vegan 29, 49, 69, 94

Vegetables 29, 32, 38, 42, 44-46, 85

Vegetarian 48, 69

Vitamins 15, 37, 41, 51-52

W

Wheat 38, 87, 106-107, 233

Y

Yeast 21

Printed in Great Britain
by Amazon